Lose weight and stay slim

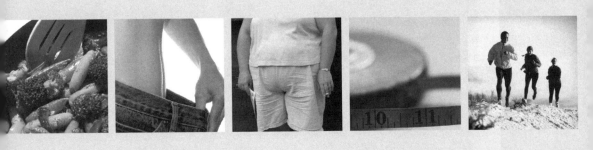

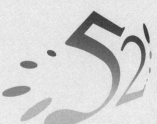

brilliantideas

one good idea can change your life...

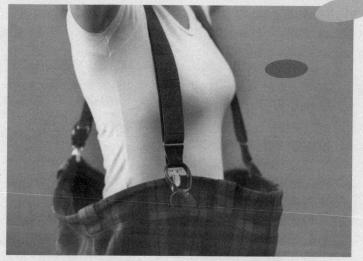

Lose weight and stay slim

Secrets of fad-free dieting

Eve Cameron

Careful now

It's your life so be sensible about how you take care of it. You should consult your doctor or healthcare provider before changing your diet, undergoing any kind of change to your exercise routine or taking any nutritional supplements.

If you have any health problems of any nature – physical, emotional or mental – always consult the proper healthcare providers.

First published in 2005 by
The Infinite Ideas Company Limited
Belsyre Court
57 Woodstock Road
Oxford
OX2 6HJ
United Kingdom
www.infideas.com

CIP catalogue records for this book are available from the British Library and the US Library of Congress.

ISBN 1-904902-22-7

Brand and product names are trademarks or registered trademarks of their respective owners.

Designed and typeset by Baseline Arts Ltd, Oxford
Printed and bound by TJ International, Cornwall

Brilliant ideas

Brilliant features

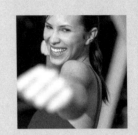

Each chapter of this book is designed to provide you with an inspirational idea that you can read quickly and put into practice straight away.

Throughout you'll find four features that will help you to get right to the heart of the idea:

- *Try another idea* If this idea looks like a life-changer then there's no time to lose. *Try another idea* will point you straight to a related tip to expand and enhance the first.

- *Here's an idea for you* Give it a go – right here, right now – and get an idea of how well you're doing so far.

- *Defining ideas* Words of wisdom from masters and mistresses of the art, plus some interesting hangers-on.

- *How did it go?* If at first you do succeed try to hide your amazement. If, on the other hand, you don't this is where you'll find a Q and A that highlights common problems and how to get over them.

Introduction

I swear it appeared overnight. That spare tyre around my middle was not there when I was thirty-four. But on my thirty-fifth birthday I saw it hanging over my jeans.

I tried holding my tummy in. I tried walking taller. I tried on a different pair of jeans. But there it sat, like a hideous unwanted gift that you haven't got the receipt for, so can't take back. I knew perfectly well how it had got there though. Despite being a regular exerciser, I was also a big eater. As well as consuming large portions of food, I had, and still have actually, a Very Sweet Tooth, so I'd have lots of sweet things as snacks too. At some point, the calories in must have overtaken the calories out, which is how I, and in fact how anyone, puts on weight. Yes, there may be other reasons (medications and medical conditions for example) but mostly you gain weight because you eat too much and don't move enough. So, the solution is quite obviously to eat less and move more. But of course that's easier said than done. Still, there's plenty of help out there. Isn't there?

Does the world really need another diet book I asked myself when I first spoke to Infinite Ideas. If it didn't, we decided, we'd all be slim, healthy and happy, because all those other diet books would have answered our questions, given us all the advice and tips we need and the motivation and success tools to help us lose weight and, importantly, keep it off. So, what's different about this book? First, there's the fabulous format. The chapters, or ideas, as we prefer to call them, are nice, manageable chunks, that are self-contained, yet link to other ideas. Each also has a section that answers the questions you might have on a given subject. This format means you can dip in and out as you please, though if you want to read the whole book in one go, do feel free.

Content-wise, rather than being the sort of diet book that tells you to have 50 g of pineapple for lunch, or to do fifty press ups before breakfast, you'll find that this is a more holistic guide to losing weight. It deals with motivation, body shape, healthy eating, decoding food labels, fitness and examines popular diets and much more! In short, it's packed with everything that could possibly be relevant to you and losing weight.

Throughout the book, you'll find some recurring themes, which I think are the key issues of successful weight loss. And because they're key issues, I'm going to tell you what they are here (but I hope you still read the rest of the book).

Diets are not something to be jumped on and off like buses. That's why most diets don't work. A special diet may be fine (unless you get really bored by day three) until you go back to eating normally and then you pile the pounds back on. The only way to lose weight permanently is to change your eating habits for good. That doesn't mean denial either (most diets are about denial by the way) – it's about eating healthily, consuming a variety of foods, some in moderation and keeping a check on your portion sizes. Small changes and a long-term view are more successful than short-term bursts of enthusiasm.

Physical activity is a must. That doesn't mean that you have to work out at a gym with muscle-bound Vin Diesel look-alikes every night of the week. But what it does mean is getting at least half an hour's moderate exercise five times a week. It could be gym-based, studio classes, sports, dancing, running, walking – anything really to get your heart rate up and work those muscles. As well as burning up calories and toning your body, exercise has so many health benefits, it's worth making time for it. And if you have kids, make activity part of their lives too, for fun, but also for their future health and wellbeing.

Realistic goals are essential for motivation and success. There are tools in this book to help you work out whether you really are overweight and by how much. But it's important to be realistic in your goals. A small, apple-shaped person can never be a tall pear-shaped person and vice versa. Aim to be in the best possible shape you can be. If you set yourself achievable targets you'll get there. Goals that are impossible to reach just make you miserable. Equally, be realistic about the speed at which you'll lose weight. Crash diets (which are faddy diets or very low calorie ones) cause rapid weight loss, but it's mostly water and lean tissue, rather than fat. Eating sensibly and losing just a pound or two a week is preferable – it's easier for one thing, not to mention healthier for your body and most important of all is sustainable, i.e. you won't suddenly return to your former weight the minute you so much as look at a doughnut. Remember, the tortoise won the race, not the hare!

So those are the big learning points, but this book gives you all the knowledge, tips and ideas you'll need in bite-sized chunks that will get you to where you want to be. And if there's one other suggestion I could make, it's cook, or learn to cook! Most experts now agree that part of our burgeoning obesity problem is due to the fact that we rely on junk food, takeaways and processed, ready-made meals. Home-made food tends to be lower in fat, salt and sugar (and of course contains fewer additives). I found myself agreeing with Prince Charles recently, who was saying how he thought domestic science should be reintroduced to schools. Most kids I know don't have a clue how to boil an egg. In fact, lots of grown ups I know don't know how to boil an egg! The truth is it takes the same amount of time to whip up a tasty, healthy, weight-loss-friendly meal as it does to reheat a ready meal or get a takeaway. The price isn't that different either. The only difference is to your waistline. Do you think the world could use another cookbook?

Here's to your success!

Eve

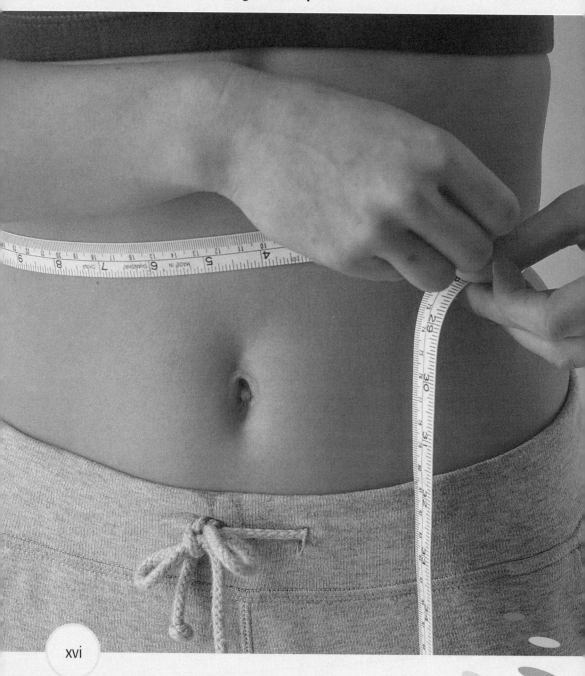

1

A weighty issue (or, a weighty question)

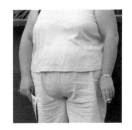

Have your waistbands been feeling a little tighter recently? Or are kaftans the only clothes you really feel comfortable in now? Here's how to work out roughly the right weight for you, plus some news you can use about body shape.

Judging by the newspaper headlines screaming about some new statistic or research about obesity, you'd think there was a moral obligation to be thin.

Often the subtext is that fat people get sick and are a burden on our medical resources. And then there are the images of super-slim models and celebrities that confront us in magazines and on our TV and movie screens. The underlying message here is that this is the way you're supposed to look, especially if you want to be happy and successful, not to mention being sexually attractive. Yet half the world is starving. It's enough to make you choke on your chocolate bar, isn't it?

Measure your waist and hips. Many experts are now saying that abdominal fat is the killer, with apple-shaped people who have relatively slim hips and a larger waist being more at risk from developing heart disease than the pear-shaped – those who carry their fat on their hips and thighs. The ideal waist measurement for men is less than 95 cm (37 inches) and less than 80 cm (32 inches) for women. Over 100 cm (40 inches) for a man and over 90 cm (35 inches) for a woman indicates the greatest risk to health.

Obesity is undeniably a growing problem in the Western world, due mainly to the over-consumption of the wrong kinds of foods and decreased activity levels. Experts warn of the host of health dangers to which carrying too much weight exposes you, including heart disease, diabetes, high blood pressure and, for women in particular (though not exclusively), fertility problems. It's not guaranteed that you'll develop these kinds of health problems – obesity just heightens your risk, which is of course why most of us just carry on regardless – until something goes wrong. The chances are that if you're already suffering any of the conditions mentioned, your doctor has grilled you on your diet and suggested losing weight.

For the majority of us, slimming down is more of a preventative health measure or something we want to do for cosmetic reasons: i.e. we just don't like the way we look. This is fine, as long as it isn't interfering with daily life and manifesting itself as disordered eating (anorexia, bulimia, faddy eating and so on). If that is the case for you, please seek help through a doctor or therapist. Life is too short and too precious not to enjoy it to the full.

Working out if you're really overweight is easily done using the Body Mass Index calculation. I have to point out that this method is not without its critics (partly because if you're quite well-muscled, you'll be heavy, not fat, because muscle weighs more than fat) but my feeling is you have to start somewhere! All you have to do is weigh yourself and record the result in kilograms. Then measure your height in metres. Then do the following sum:

If you're doubtful or put off by the idea of more physical activity, turn to IDEA 12, Why exercise makes you feel on top of the world.

Try another idea…

weight in kilograms divided by (height in metres × height in metres) = BMI

Example:
You weigh 70 kg and you are 1.6 metres tall

'I'm not overweight. I'm just nine inches too short.'
SHELLEY WINTERS

Defining idea…

$$70 \div (1.6 \times 1.6) =$$
$$70 \div 2.56 = 27.34$$
$$BMI = 27.34$$

Check your own result against the ranges below

BMI for men	BMI for women	
Under 20	under 19	underweight
20–24.9	19–24.9	normal
25–29.9	25–29.9	overweight
30 plus	30 plus	obese

I fall into the upper level of normal weight, which is fine from a fatness perspective, but I know that I've crept up two dress sizes in the past decade and so estimate that losing three kilos (and keeping it off!) would take me where I want to be. That's my weight-loss mission; now work out yours.

How did it go?

Q   But I come from a fat family. I don't stand a chance...do I?

A   *We can blame our parents for lots of things, including a tendency to gain weight. However, much of 'hereditary' weight gain can also be explained by learned behaviour. For instance, if you come from a family that loves food, over-eating may be part of your lifestyle, but habits can be unlearned.*

Q   Could my weight gain be a result of a slow metabolism?

A   *Your BMR, or basal metabolic rate, is the number of calories your body needs to maintain its vital functions. This is partly to do with genetic inheritance. A friend who is a similar height and weight to you may well be able to eat more than you and not gain weight. This is very annoying, but you're probably better at other things than he or she is. There are two things to remember. First, if you have less body fat and more muscle, your metabolism will be higher, as muscle burns up more calories than fat. That's why including exercise in your weight loss plan really works. Second, don't try to cut calories drastically, as your metabolic rate will slow to adjust – and you'll just feel hungry all the time. Eating less but eating well is the key to long-term weight loss.*

Q   Why is it that men can eat more than women?

A   *The reason is that they are mostly bigger than women, so they use more energy for day-to-day maintenance. They also tend to have more lean muscle tissue than women – muscle tissue is more metabolically active than fat tissue, which means it uses up more energy (calories) to exist. Women tend to have more fat tissue.*

2

Food accountancy
made simple

You can eat them, count them or ignore them, but here's why knowing your calories from your onions is the key to losing weight.

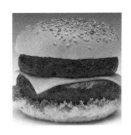

Many books make calories unnecessarily hard to understand, but the concept is really quite simple. Once you have grasped what calories mean, you have a powerful tool to help you control your weight.

Put simply, calories are just the basic units by which both the energy values of food and the energy needs of the body are measured.

You may be familiar with diets that advocate counting your daily calorie intake. It's now seen as a rather old-fashioned way to slim, not least because you have to weigh things obsessively and eating anywhere but at home becomes a nightmare. It can also make you very boring to be around as you proceed to tot up the number of calories on everyone's plate. You may find that friends stop returning your calls!

Include soya products in your diet. A particular isoflavone in soya may hold the key to improving the rate at which your cells burn up fat. It also boosts your metabolism slightly and reduces your appetite. From a looks perspective, I have it on good authority that soya helps to make your nails grow too!

However, it is really important to have some general knowledge about the calorific value of foods so you can make the best choices about what you're going to eat.

Most foods are a combination of protein, fat and carbohydrate in different ratios depending on the food. Gram for gram, fat contains 9 calories, protein and carbohydrates 4 calories and alcohol, if you're interested, 7 calories. Basically if you eat anything in excess, there's the potential that it will be more than your body needs in terms of energy or calories and will end up stored as fat. Of course it's easier to reach your maximum calorie needs quickly if you cram in lots of high-fat foods, as they have the most calories. Also, the most nutritious choices may not always be available, especially when you are away from home.

HOW MANY CALORIES DO YOU NEED?

I'm going to give you a basic formula to work this out (calculators at the ready!) but it will only be an approximate calculation. It should still be enlightening, though. The reason it is only an approximation is because if we were going to be really scientific, we would have to factor in other information. Your gym or local health centre can probably help you with these calculations if you want to be more precise.

'Two out of every three men in the UK are now classed as overweight or obese.'
THE BRITISH DIETETIC ASSOCIATION

One of the factors that makes a difference is your age, because your calorie needs diminish as you get older. By the way, this is for adults only, so please don't try this on your kids. Your sex is important too. As men have more muscle than women and muscle burns up more calories than fat, men need more calories just to exist.

Understanding the nutritional values of what you eat is vital. Wise up with IDEA 30, *What does it say on the label?*

Try another idea...

Now let's play with some numbers:

First work out your *basal metabolic rate* (BMR) which tells you the energy you need to stay alive. Multiply your weight in pounds by 10 if you're a woman, or 11 if you're a man. (If you're a metric sort of person, first multiply your weight in kilos by 2.2 to get the poundage.) Next, factor in how active you are by multiplying the sum above by 0.2 if you only do very light activities, by 0.3 if you do a little more formal exercise such as walking as well as housework, by 0.4 if you are moderately active and you rarely sit still or by 0.5 if your job involves manual labour or you play lots of sports. The result is the number of calories you need on top of your BMR.

'If you are going to lose weight and avoid gaining it, eating less is more effective than exercise alone... Doing both is the most effective combination.'
Sir JOHN KREBS, Chair of the Food Standards Agency

Defining idea...

Eating and digesting food uses up around 10% of your calorie needs, so, after adding your BMR and the extra calories you worked out for your activity levels together, work out what 10% is. Now add all three of those figures together and you'll have the number of your total calorie needs per day.

To lose half a kilo (a pound) a week, you need to cut your daily calories by 500 (or cut fewer than that and make up the difference with exercise), which is a safe amount to aim for. Although this might not sound a lot, it's easier to achieve in the long term and easier to sustain. If you lose lots of weight very quickly, you're more likely to put it back on and get into that yo-yo dieting spiral.

OK, end of accountancy lesson. Who'd have thought that playing with numbers could be such fun!

How did it go?

Q   Couldn't I just cut my calories to make the weight fall off?

A   *You could, but it's not a smart thing to do. This kind of crash dieting means that water and protein are lost from the body rather than fat. Your metabolic rate will also slow to conserve calories. As soon as you eat normally, you'll gain weight. For this reason, you really shouldn't go below 1200 calories a day. If you take the long-term view and lose weight slowly, you'll still lose water to begin with, but you'll soon start making a dent in your fat reserves, which is what you really want. Losing weight slowly with an accompanying change in lifestyle is the recipe for long-term success.*

Q   Surely if I eat high calorie foods, I could just burn off the excess with exercise?

A   *In principle I suppose you could eat rubbish and run it off. The trouble is that you could end up malnourished if this is your long-term diet tactic. Many high-fat foods don't offer enough of a nutritional balance to subsist on. Equally, even if you ran off the calories from, say, a daily ham, egg and cheese quiche, the saturated fat could still have an effect on your cholesterol levels. So, it's better to have a balanced diet with plenty of variety for your health and weight.*

3

Setting goals (without always having to move the goalposts)

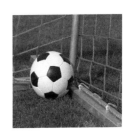

Master the art of goal-setting to turn your dream of losing weight into reality. Most of us don't do it, but planning really works!

A well-known study of a group of US students in the 1950s found that only three per cent of the graduates wrote a set of goals for their lives.

A follow-up survey some twenty years later discovered that the goal-setting students were worth more financially than the other 97% put together. You may say, well, life's not all about money. No, it's not – but the goal setters were also healthier and happier in their relationships than the others.

Goal-setting is as relevant to weight loss as it is to life plans, but it's not always as straightforward as it seems. Simply saying 'I want to lose weight' may well be true and seem to be a goal, but it won't get you very far. Why? Because goals need to be SMART:

Here's an idea for you...

Write your goals down and pin them up in a place where you will see them every day, like the fridge door. When you look at them, repeat them to yourself and visualise how you will look and feel when you have achieved them. This will keep your goals real and alive.

that's Specific, Measurable, Attainable, Realistic and Time-framed. Put simply, by analysing how to reach your end goal, you increase your chances of achieving it.

OK, let's do it. Get some paper and a pen and start writing.

Be Specific – Write down how much weight you want to lose. Is there also a particular reason you want to lose this amount, for a special occasion, or is it for health reasons? Perhaps you've always been overweight and really want to do something about it. It's important to think around the reasons you want to slim down as part of the 'why' of your goal. Once it's clear in your head, you'll be in control and focused.

Measurable – How will you measure you weight loss? By weighing yourself regularly or by dropping a clothing size? Or will you just go by the way you look or feel? How often will you take stock of your achievements? There's no right or wrong answer here – it's just about what works for you.

Attainable – Question yourself as to whether this goal is really what you want. You could think about it in terms of your commitment and enthusiasm. If you're not 100% happy about your goal, maybe you need to revisit the specifics to review whether it is too ambitious or too challenging for you to feel confident about it. A goal does have to stretch you, but if it seems unattainable you'll become downhearted pretty quickly. Of course, we all have different definitions of what's attainable and what isn't – it depends on factors such as your personality, confidence and experience.

Realistic – With the best will in the world, if you are 165 cm (5 ft 5 in) and pear-shaped, no diet is going to turn you into Aussie model/actress/business woman Elle McPherson – especially if you're a man! Make sure your goal is realistic. Think about your goal in terms of being the best you can be.

Setting goals is a major step in slimming successfully. You can take it further by developing it like a formal business plan. Turn to IDEA 5, *Learn to act like the chief executive of You Inc.* for inspiration.

Try another idea...

Time-framed – A time frame keeps your goal on track. Set a start point, such as 'I will start my healthy eating weight loss plan on Thursday' and give yourself an end time too, such as 'I will lose five kilos by my summer holiday.' I think it also makes sense to include a couple of time frames in your overall goal representing short and longer term achievements. This helps with motivation. So you could add 'I will start exercising three times a week on Mondays, Wednesdays and Saturdays from next week' and so on. Use positive goal-getting language when writing down what you're going to achieve. There's no room here for 'might' and 'ought to'.

By now your goal should be looking so clear that you can reach out and touch it. I hope you feel all revved up and ready to go. One other thing: do remember to congratulate yourself every step of the way, whether it is with little (non-fattening) rewards or simply a mental pat on the back.

'To begin with the end in mind means to start with a clear understanding of your destination.'
STEPHEN COVEY

Defining idea...

How did it go?

Q My goals seem a bit confused. How can I make them clearer?

A Maybe you're just very good at listing what you don't want in life! You may need to work a bit harder on identifying what you really do want. You need to be clear about this in order to make it happen.

Q What if I mess up and don't achieve my goals?

A Come on, do you know anyone who does everything perfectly all the time? Everyone messes up. Learn from your mistakes, move on and try again.

Q How much weight could I aim to lose per week?

A The ideal weight-loss pattern needs to be long-term and sustainable. If you crash diet, by dramatically reducing the number of calories you take in, you will lose more weight initially (though this won't all be fat), but you will soon plateau, as your body slows down to cope with what it sees as starvation. The end result is that you will be terribly hungry most of the time and as soon as you start to eat normally you will put weight back on. To lose half a kilo (a pound) a week, you need to shed 500 calories a day on average. That means eating a bit less and/or exercising more. And that's not really too hard. Trust me!

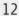

4

Pyramid selling

What's a healthy balance of foods? Get to grips with the basics and you're halfway to being slim – eating better becomes much easier when you are clear about this.

One of the cleverest tools to help you to keep to a balanced diet has to be the food guide pyramid, first conceived in the USA.

The food guide pyramid is a simple way of visualising the kinds of foods to eat and the proportions in which we need them for a healthy diet. The pyramid is a standard for health, and it is incredibly useful for dieters as you can still use its principles, but just eat less. An added bonus is that the more you know about food, the greater your chances of slimming successfully.

It's important to be reminded that eating a variety of foods is considered essential for optimum health. By eating as the pyramid suggests, you should get your protein, vitamins, minerals and fibre, without overdoing the fat, cholesterol, sugars, salt and calories! Each group in the pyramid has a suggested amount of servings attached to it, with the lowest number intended for people consuming 1600 calories a day, such as sedentary women, while the highest number is intended for people

Here's an idea for you...

If you're not keen on pyramid shapes, try a circle, split into the following segments, as suggested by the UK Food Standards Agency: 30% fruit and veg, 30% bread, pasta, rice and potatoes, 15% dairy, 15% meat and fish, and 10% fat and sugary foods. These are the proportions you need for a balanced diet.

needing around 2800 calories a day, such as male manual labourers. The large differences in calorie needs have confused some people, so right now the Americans are working on making it clearer. As long as you remember to look to the lower levels, you'll be doing well!

The food pyramid works like this. At the bottom of the pyramid, the wide base, you'll find the bread, cereal, rice and pasta group, of which the recommended intake is 6–11 servings. Moving up a layer are the fruits and vegetables, with a little more emphasis on vegetables, with 3–5 servings recommended and 2–4 of fruit. The next layer of the pyramid is for milk, yoghurt and cheese (dairy products), but excluding butter and cream and, sharing the space on this tier, is the group featuring meat, fish, dry beans, eggs and nuts. You should aim for 2–3 servings per day from each of these groups. Then at the top, in the tiny space at the pyramid's summit, is the fats, oils and sweets group, with the caution 'use sparingly'.

As an exercise, compare the pyramid with your daily or weekly food intake. How does your diet shape up? The vast majority of people in the Western world have diets that turn the pyramid on its head, with fats and sugars making up the bulk of their food consumption.

By this point you may feel as though your head is exploding, but I have to tell you one more thing: within each of the groups there are healthier and more diet-friendly choices to be made. For example, in the cereals group, choose wholemeal, brown or unrefined products because they give you more fibre, vitamins and minerals. In principle cakes such as muffins and croissants belong in this group, but they bring more fat and sugar to the party than anything really nutritionally interesting.

As well as what you eat, how you prepare it counts too. See IDEA 23, *Make your kitchen more diet-friendly.*

Try another idea...

You can't go far wrong with fruit and vegetables, apart from serving them up with cream, butter or deep-frying them! Frozen and canned fruit and vegetables count too, but with canned produce check that what you're buying doesn't contain added sugar or salt. Wherever possible choose lower fat versions of dairy products and watch out for creamy dishes. With meats, look for lean cuts or trim off any visible fat; for example, chicken is much less fatty if you remove the skin. Avoid processed meat products as far as possible, as they tend to be very fatty. Fish is mostly lean, apart from oily fish such as fresh tuna, mackerel and salmon. However these contain the omega-3 essential fatty acids which have great health benefits, such as reducing the risk of death from heart disease. You should definitely aim for two portions of oily fish a week.

'I do not like broccoli. And I haven't liked it since I was a little kid and my mother made me eat it. And I'm President of the United States and I'm not going to eat any more broccoli.'
GEORGE BUSH, SENIOR

Defining idea...

How did it go?

Q   I'm not keen on meat. Is there a vegetarian pyramid?

A   Yes and it's pretty similar to the original. Soya, nuts, seeds and legumes replace meat and are actually a great alternative to meat for carnivores who want to ring the changes. The wide base of the pyramid is a mix of fruit and vegetables, whole grains and legumes. These should be eaten at every meal. You have to watch getting overly dependent on eggs and hard cheese, because as well as being a source of protein they are high in fat and should only be eaten occasionally. Nuts and seeds should be eaten daily as they are highly nutritious, but only in very small quantities (a small handful) as they are fat-rich too.

Q   What group does something like a burger fall into?

A   If it's between two bits of roll and has salad added, it contains meat, cereal and vegetable. Many dishes are a combination of the food groups.

Q   I don't eat much fish, but I do eat canned tuna – does that count as oily fish?

A   Fresh tuna counts as oily fish but canned tuna does not. In the canning process, the omega-3 benefits are lost. However, canned tuna is still a good source of protein. Make sure you buy it in spring water though, to avoid adding extra fat in the form of oils used in canning or salt, which is added when it is canned in brine.

5

Learn to act like the chief executive of You Inc.

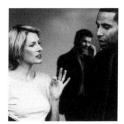

You wouldn't run a business or a household without a plan, especially if big changes were looming. As the person in charge of your mind and body, try this life coaching technique to develop your successful slimming strategy.

I first got interested in life coaching when I wasn't happy in my life, but wasn't sure what was really wrong. Going on a coaching course helped me to focus my thoughts with amazing clarity.

I ended up quitting my job as a magazine editor and became a freelance editor and writer, reinventing and rediscovering my life along the way. But enough about me! My point to you is that wanting to lose weight is a serious business and like any of life's challenges, it can be fraught with confusion, doubts, false starts and questions. A proper game plan can iron out many issues you'll face along the way, hence this introduction to a really useful life coaching exercise (and at a fraction of the price of a course!).

Here's an idea for you...

There's nothing like a declutter to rev up your energy and motivation levels. Try one or all of these for your fresh start:

- **Clean out your fridge and cupboards and get rid of diet saboteurs such as the deep fat fryer and the biscuit tin.**

- **Go through your wardrobe and bag up all the clothes you haven't worn for a year and are unlikely to wear again.**

- **Give yourself a new haircut or a beauty/grooming treatment. Make yourself feel good.**

The GROW model stands for Goals, Reality, Options and Will. Grab a piece of paper and write those headings down leaving enough space to add your thoughts and answers beneath them:

Goals – I know that you are reading this book because your goal is to lose weight, but you need to break that goal down to make it achievable. Go for specifics, such as 'I want to lose three kilos by my wedding day' or 'I want to be my target weight by my holiday'. As well as making your goal realistic and positive, give it a time frame. Also, write down why you want lose weight. Is it for health reasons, for instance? Or is it about your self-esteem? Reminding yourself why you want to lose weight reinforces that goal.

Reality – Think about your weight now. How much control do you have over reducing it? What are the main obstacles you see that could prevent you from losing weight? What resources do you have that will help you? Maybe you have inner resources, such as a determination to succeed that you've demonstrated in your career, or perhaps you have a great municipal leisure centre near you or a corporate gym membership through your workplace. Think about what else could help you achieve your goal and who else you could ask for help.

Options – OK, now you really have to free up your mind to think laterally and creatively! Write down all the ways you think you could approach your weight loss (following the ideas in this book should be on your list, but add your own thoughts) When you've come to the end of your list, write down some more ideas, even if they seem silly or far-fetched. If you're stuck, think about what you might advise a friend if he or she wanted to slim down. If time and money were unlimited, what might you do then? Do you know anyone who has recently lost weight? How did they do it? How would you feel if you didn't lose weight?

Positive encouragement from friends, family and fellow dieters will help you to stay motivated and make the process easier. Why not join a slimming club? See IDEA 28, Members only.

Try another idea...

Will – Looking at your options, write down the ones that appeal to you and which could take you part or all of the way to your final goal. Think about the obstacles you could face if you chose any of those options. Here's another hard bit. When are you going start? Are you fully committed to seeing this through? Give yourself a mark on a scale of 1–10.

'If you can dream it, you can do it.'
WALT DISNEY

Defining idea...

Well done! You've completed your self-coaching exercise and should have a clearer framework about what you want to achieve and how you're going to get there. May be it threw up other areas in your life which need attention, in which case, follow the same process through, substituting the issue. All for no extra charge!

'Imagination is more important than knowledge.'
ALBERT EINSTEIN

Defining idea...

19

How did it go?

Q **I've tried losing weight before and just can't seem to do it. How can I make it different this time?**

A *Have you ever heard of a self-fulfilling prophecy? What you think is what you get, so work on your beliefs about what you can achieve, rather than what you think you can't. Use positive self-talk. You could start by rephrasing the negative attitude above to say, 'I have tried losing weight before and have learned a lot about how not to do it.'*

Q **I have so many responsibilities in my life that I usually come last on the list. How can I find the time?**

A *Go back to the reality section of the GROW model exercise and make a list of all the obstacles and all those other responsibilities in your life that may prevent you achieving your goal of weight loss. There are always solutions to issues, whether that means rethinking your childcare arrangements, working different hours, going to bed earlier so you can wake up earlier to go to the gym, preparing yourself a healthy packed lunch, asking your partner to do more around the house and so on. Think hard, think long, think laterally and ask someone else to help think with you. You could also probably learn to say 'no' more often. Don't be a martyr.*

6

Get the write habit

Why keeping a diary helps you lose weight.

Noting down what you are eating may give you some surprises. It will definitely help you to identify the changes you need to make to help you to lose weight.

All too often we're not realistic about what and how much we really eat. Sometimes we truly forget. Check how often you're eating, too.

Sometimes we're in denial and it's simply easier to forget, to assuage feelings of guilt, self-loathing or defeatism (all common negative attitudes when you're trying to lose weight). Keeping a record of your food and drink consumption is an invaluable tool when you're starting out on a weight loss plan, as it gives you a real insight into the kinds of foods you usually eat and the quantity and frequency of meals and snacks. Unless you know where you're going wrong, how can you put things right? The food diary doesn't lie – unless you cheat, of course. All you have to do is record faithfully everything you eat and drink for a week. That includes the 'I

Here's an idea for you... **Visualisation techniques are used by high achievers in many demanding fields such as sport and business. It is a proven psychological method of helping you to attain your goals. For a few minutes every day, picture yourself achieving your goals and how you'll feel and look when you've achieved them. Don't laugh – it works for Olympic gold medal winners!**

nibbled such a small piece of cheese that I'm sure it doesn't count' snacks and the croissant (so full of fat!) that you grabbed on your way to work. If you ate it while you were walking, it doesn't mean you didn't eat it. Equally, don't try to change your eating habits temporarily to appear more virtuous, as you'll miss the benefits of the exercise.

At the end of the week, take time to really study your diary and ask yourself the following questions:

■ Am I eating regularly (breakfast, lunch and dinner)?

Skipping proper meals is not a good way to lose weight. You'll probably compensate by over-eating at the next one or indulging in high-calorie, fat-laden, quick-fix snacks when you're suddenly ravenous.

■ How often am I eating between meals and what am I grazing on?

This could be because you are skipping meals, or are you are snacking a lot as well as eating regular meals? If those in-between snacks are fundamentally healthy, such as fruit or low-fat yoghurt, then that's OK, but if they are more likely to be crisps and bars of chocolate or an entire packet of biscuits (hey, I've done it!), you'll simply be taking in more calories than you need. The result? Weight gain.

■ Is my diet sufficiently varied? Does your diary tell you that you're eating the same foods day in, day out? And what types of food are they?

We need a variety of foods for optimum health as well as keeping our taste buds interested. Check the mix in your meals. Do they include a variety of different food groups on a daily basis? Very broadly, we need proteins (meat, fish, eggs, pulses, beans) carbohydrates (bread, cereal, pasta, rice, potatoes) and plenty of fruit and vegetables, plus some fats and dairy produce.

Make notes in your food diary of what you're feeling when you eat. It could be that sometimes you're eating because you're bored or feeling unhappy. If this sounds familiar, try reading IDEA 14, Are you an emotional eater?

Try another idea...

■ Do I rely on junk food, take-aways and ready-prepared meals?

Our lives are busy, but if you eat this way all the time, weight gain is inevitable due to the high fat and calorie content of these types of food. You can improve on convenience and fast foods by serving your own vegetables or salads as an accompaniment. Cooking from scratch gives you the ultimate control over exactly what goes in to your food. It doesn't have to be expensive, difficult or time-consuming. Buy yourself a low-fat cook book and impress yourself.

'My doctor told me to stop having intimate dinners for four. Unless there are three other people.'
ORSON WELLES

Defining idea...

■ What am I drinking?

Consider your alcohol consumption. If you drink it, are you within the recommended health guidelines? The recommended maximum is 21 units of alcohol a week for a man and 14 units for a woman Seen from a dieting perspective, alcohol is just empty calories. Do you drink lots of fizzy drinks? Some contain up to seven teaspoons of sugar. Fruit juice, although 'natural' and seemingly good for you, also contains lots of sugars which, if you're downing a litre a day, adds up to a lot of extra calories too. Are you drinking enough water? Are you drinking any water at all? Our bodies need water to help the absorption of nutrients from food. When you're properly hydrated, you'll feel and see other benefits too.

Now make a list of what you could change and how you'll do it. Start with the simplest changes and implement them quickly so you'll feel encouraged.

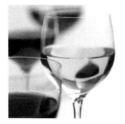
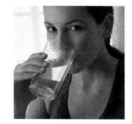
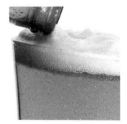

Q   **I'm too busy to write things down and besides at the end of the day I can't remember what I've had. How am I going to keep my food diary up to date?**

How did it go?

A   *The idea of a food diary may seem pedantic, but research shows that people who keep these records are more likely to lose weight. Rather than trying to recall everything at the end of the day, get a little notebook and write details as you go. If you whip your diary out before you consume something, it gives you a moment to really consider your food choices too.*

Q   **In my job I have to eat out a lot. How can you expect me to control my diet, let alone keep a diary?**

A   *That's a great excuse! The occasional meal out and eating what you fancy is fine, and if you do have to eat out a lot, you need to make the best choices from what is available. That means saying no to creamy sauces and anything fried. Choose a salad as a starter with a light vinaigrette rather than heavy dressings like Thousand Island or mayonnaise. Choose a fruit salad for dessert, not a sticky toffee pudding with extra cream. Say yes to grills and anything steamed and keep sauces and dressings on the side so you can control how much you add, which will be just a spoonful or two, won't it?*

25

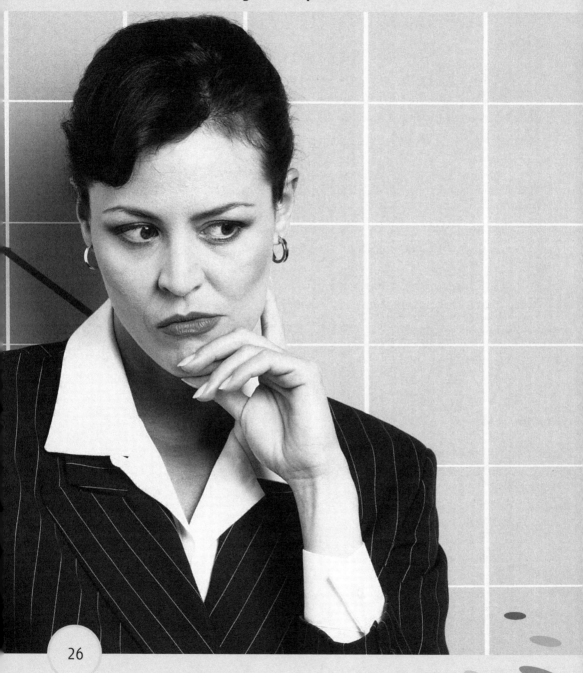

7

It's never too late to change your mind

Have you been on diets before, lost weight, then regained it and lost motivation? Change your attitude to dieting and use your mind to get ahead.

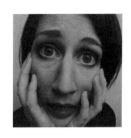

I have a friend who's been on every kind of diet going: cabbage soup, high protein, eating for your blood type, meal replacements and all the rest. The trouble is, she hasn't changed her poor mental attitude to dieting.

She uses diets like buses, jumping on and off. If she's just missed one, well, there will be another along in a minute, won't there? Has she lost weight? Yes, she has and then she's gained it, until the next period of dieting when the cycle repeats itself.

Why is it that most diets only seem to work temporarily? In my opinion the main reason is that they don't teach you much about healthy eating or help you learn a healthy attitude to food. All too often, entire food groups are banned, which,

Here's an idea for you...

Drink fruit juice not cola. According to new research from the American Diabetes Association, just one regular can of a fizzy drink a day is enough to increase your risk of diabetes by 85%. A can a day could also lead to a weight gain of around a stone in four years.

depending on the group, can be unhealthy or even dangerous if you follow it for a long time. Meal replacements, although designed nowadays to be nutritionally safe, don't really give the average dieter any idea of what a healthy meal looks like. If a diet promises you rapid weight loss, you can bet it will be due to consuming significantly less calories. It won't be because of some magical fat-burning enzyme found in the bongo-bongo fruit or whatever the angle is! Besides, you'll just lose water and lean muscle mass anyway, so it won't necessarily be sustainable.

Diets can be as dull as ditchwater, particularly if they are very strict about what you can and can't eat. Not only do you feel bored and start fantasising about bathing in jelly and custard (mmm, with some chocolate sprinkles too), but they can make eating out difficult, especially when you visit friends' houses. You have to be very good company indeed to make up for your inconvenient food requests. Let's face it, a diet can simply be hard to fit into your life, particularly when you also have a family to feed or if you work long or unusual hours. And then there's the hunger, the growling stomach and the faintness-inducing pangs that all too often lead to a binge. Then you feel guilty – and move on to another diet in the hope that it will be better.

Many people who sincerely want to lose weight are failing to stick to their diet regimes. So what does work? There isn't one single way to lose weight successfully. You need to develop a combination of tricks that work for you, and an acceptance of certain key points. The first is that you will probably need to change your idea of what a diet and losing weight is all about. The kinds of diets mentioned above are not going to help you. To lose weight and keep it off, you have to change your eating habits and lifestyle permanently. Before you shriek that this sounds even scarier than a wasp-chewing diet, remember that losing weight is about the long haul, not dieting in short four-week bursts. There are no quick fixes, but if you make small changes over a period of time, they will add up to big results.

Still hankering after a quick-fix? What about the beauty creams that claim to help you lose inches? See IDEA 27, *Can beauty products help you slim?*

Try another idea...

Next, you have to realistic about your weight-loss goals. Aim to be in the best shape you can be, which is to be healthy, not to look like a stick insect. Eat a balanced selection of foods with plenty of fruit and vegetables, protein and carbohydrate and a little fat. A balanced diet is essential for good health, keeps things interesting for you and ensures you won't suffer endless cravings because you're denying yourself certain foods. Remember that you do need to keep a check on the portion sizes. You'll also be doing yourself a big favour if you become more physically active. Exercise makes you feel and look good, helps to control your appetite and, in conjunction with sensible eating, helps you lose weight faster. Using these guidelines, weight should come off slowly but surely, without you feeling as though you've put your entire life on hold to accommodate a short-term diet. You might just enjoy yourself too!

'I never worry about diets. The only carrots that interest me are the number you get in a diamond.'
MAE WEST

Defining idea...

Q **If I'm not following a strict diet where certain foods are forbidden, can I eat junk food and whatever else I like?**

A   *Whoa! Steady on. There's a big difference between having a bit of what you fancy and winning an award for being the most regular customer at the burger bar. The key is to make fattening, less healthy foods an occasional treat rather than your regular diet and to choose small portions. That way, you don't feel deprived. Be flexible in your approach. If you eat sensibly most of the time, the odd blow-out really isn't going to make much difference.*

Q **How can I stop feeling hungry all the time?**

A   *Try using this mental trick to manipulate your appetite: visualise a dial that represents your hunger, on a scale from zero to ten. Eight to ten is ravenous, five to seven is hungry, below five is not very hungry. At the moment, where does the dial have to be for you to eat? Perhaps it's hovering around four, in which case you need to set it a little higher, so you're only eating when you're really hungry. Reset your dial in your imagination, perhaps to six to begin with. Every time you're about to eat something, see your dial and stop to ask yourself where you are on it hunger-wise. Over a period of time, you'll find that you've stopped eating when the dial is under five. Think before you eat and only eat when you're hungry!*

8

I'll have a 21, 34 and 52 please...oh and a large portion of 15

The road to Fatville is paved with fast food and takeaways, but you don't have to cut them out of your life completely – it's just a balancing act.

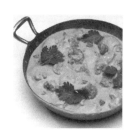

Eating takeaways and other fast foods is the norm for many of us. With little or no washing up to do, no shopping and cooking, this way of eating can feel like a life-saver for busy people.

The trouble is that when you eat fast food you have no idea what you're really consuming in terms of fat, calories, hidden salt and additives, which is bad news for your health and diet. For example, sometimes a chicken nugget is only distantly related to chickens and what you're really eating is just a load of old filler. A beefburger, fries and cola drink are one of the cultural icons of the free world, but they are also a symbol of today's fat world and can easily add up to over a thousand calories with colossal amounts of saturated fat thrown in.

Here's an idea for you... **Why not choose soup as a starter? All that liquid fills you up and means there's less room for the temptation of garlic bread with cheese and bacon or 'Death by Chocolate' fudge cake.**

It's fine to eat takeaways and fast food occasionally, but you can always make healthier less fattening choices. I think that sometimes we just get lazy about food – here are some tips for lazy people about three popular junk food staples:

FISH AND CHIPS

- The good bits: high in protein, vitamins B6 and B12, plus a few minerals.

- The bad bits: high in fat, low on fibre. If it's a big portion, you could quite easily be consuming half the daily recommended fat levels in one sitting.

- Try this: balance out your other meal of the day with a vitamin-packed salad and some low-fat protein, such as cottage cheese, skinless chicken or tuna. Or make your own fish and chips. How hard is it to stick a piece of fish under the grill? Use prepared oven chips, rather than deep-frying your own, or make potato wedges and roast them.

PIZZA

- The good bits: cheese and tomato offers protein, calcium and some vitamins.

- The bad bits: if you go for pepperoni and extra cheese, you're piling on fat.

- Try this: balance out the pizza at your next meal with a chicken casserole and lots of vegetables for low-fat protein and plenty of fibre and vitamins. Or make your own pizza using a ready-made base. My life seems too short to make my own, but if you can, feel free. Award yourself extra points if you use wholemeal flour, which gives you more fibre and other nutrients. Top it with heaps of vegetables, a little protein (for example, chicken, turkey, lean beef, tuna or tofu). Add grated cheese, which is better than lumps, for a bit of flavour and less fat.

Is it small, medium or large? Check your sense of portion control with IDEA 10, *Why size matters.*

Try another idea...

BEEFBURGER, FRIES AND A MILKSHAKE

- The good bits: high in protein, carbohydrates and calcium, plus some vitamin A, B12 and riboflavin.

- The bad bits: high in saturated fat and sodium, low in fibre, and often a good sprinkling of additives.

- Try this: redress the balance with another meal of wholemeal pasta and vegetables for fibre and vitamins. A home-made burger is easily made with lean mince. Serve it with potato wedges and salad and either leave out the bap or use half a wholemeal roll. Make a more slimming milkshake by using skimmed milk and flavoured powder.

'We were taken to a fast food café where our order was fed into a computer. Our hamburgers, made from the flesh of chemically impregnated cattle had been broiled over counterfeit charcoal and placed between slices of artificially flavoured cardboard and served by recycled juvenile delinquents.'
JEAN MICHEL CHAPEREAU, French author

Defining idea...

When you order a take-away to eat at home, follow the advice above plus the following tips for cutting down on calories and fat overload:

- Avoid anything fried and choose grilled, steamed, broiled or baked foods without cheese and creamy sauce.

- Say no to all creamy and buttery sauces. Choose tomato-based ones.

- Watch out for coconut. It seems innocuous, but it's full of saturated fat.

- If you're having a side order of rice, ask for it plain boiled.

- Leave out the side orders of garlic bread or bread and butter. If you must have bread, do as the Continentals do and have it plain.

Here's a final thought: Stop eating when you're full!

Defining idea...

'The journey of a thousand pounds begins with a single burger.'
CHRIS O'BRIEN, writer

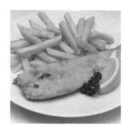
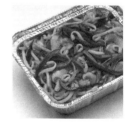

Q   **I love eating out and getting takeaways. How can I stop forgetting my good intentions and ending up hating myself?**

How did it go?

A   *If you do pig out, just get back to your sensible ways the next day. Try these points as a strategy and see if they help: skip bread or whatever snacky treat is on the table and order a couple of starters rather than a starter and a main course. You could also try sharing a dessert. Avoid anything that is described as breaded, battered, tempura, en croute or creamed and don't order dishes with fatty sauces such as béchamel, Bearnaise and Hollandaise.*

Q   **My partner and I go for an Indian or Chinese meal once a week. What are the best choices?**

A   *It's hard to avoid ghee (clarified butter) in Indian dishes, but one tip is to avoid as much sauce as you can. Creamy kormas and fried starters such as samosas and bhajis are very high in fat too, so they are best avoided. Wiser choices include tandoori chicken and prawns, grilled chicken kebabs, chicken or prawn Madras, vegetable curries, plain rice, chapattis and raita.*

At Chinese restaurants, watch out for the fattening battered or crispy dishes, such as crispy duck, prawn toast and spring rolls. Go for stir-fried and steamed food as much as possible.

35

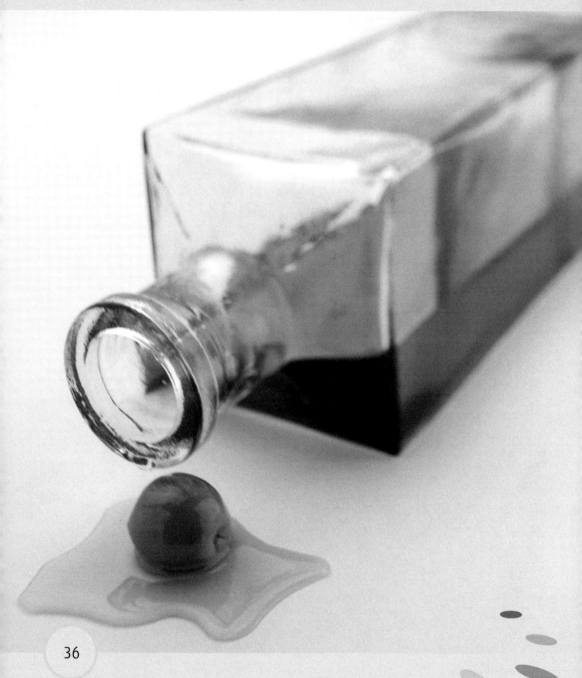

9

Fats: the good, the bad and the downright ugly

Fat friends and foes.

Eating too much of certain fats is definitely harmful to both your waistline and your health, so here are some handy hints on how to perform a bit of liposuction on your diet.

You need to know about fat in food because it's a rich source of calories. In fact, it contains more than twice as many calories, weight for weight, as carbohydrates and proteins.

As well as being a major cause of weight gain, a high-fat diet, particularly one that is high in saturated fats, can also increase your risk of heart disease and breast and bowel cancers.

Fat isn't all bad; our bodies need it. It delivers vitamins A, D, E and K and aids their absorption. It helps to regulate a variety of bodily functions. It makes food taste

Here's an
idea for
you...

Reach for your extra virgin. A drizzle a day might keep the doctor away. I use olive oil in just about everything. The trouble is that I tend to use lots of it. Yes, it's a healthy oil, but if you eat a lot of it you are just adding unnecessary calories. The key is to measure it. A tablespoon is usually enough for everything.

delicious and gives it a creamy, more-ish texture. The thing is not all fats are created equal and we typically consume too much of the wrong kind of fat and not enough of the good stuff. We should all know our rights from our wrongs for the sake of our health, but there's even more reason to get clued up when there's weight to be lost. So here are the big fat facts to chew on:

- **Saturated fats** – Foods with high levels of saturated fatty acids include butter, lard, whole milk, hard cheeses, cream, meat and meat products, palm oil and coconut oil. These are the diet wreckers and you should aim to have only a very small amount of them in your daily diet. You can reduce your intake of these kinds of fats by buying leaner cuts of meat and chopping off visible fat. Grilling, baking or steaming foods is a more slimming way to cook than smothering everything in butter and cream.

- **Trans fats** – These are found in processed foods such as crisps, cakes, biscuits and pies and also in many brands of margarine. Cross the street to avoid them. Check food labels for these fats – they'll be listed as 'hydrogenated'.

- **Unsaturated fats** – These break down into monounsaturates and polyunsaturates. Monounsaturates are found in olive oil, nut oils, avocados and seeds, which have health benefits for your heart and so are a better choice than saturated fats. But they're still fattening, so use them sparingly. Polyunsaturates pop up in most vegetable oils (corn, sunflower, safflower), fish oils and oily fish. They are generally a good thing, particularly if you consume them in place of saturated fats, although they are still calorific.

Could your lunch be piling on the pounds? Chew on IDEA 13, *Let's do lunch.*

Try another idea...

Overall, fats should make up about a third of your total daily calorie intake, with saturated fats making up less than 10% of all the calories you consume. This rule is just for general health, but as most of us consume too much fat, it should help you lose a couple of kilos. It is quite safe to cut your total intake of all types of fat to about 20% of your daily calories. To reduce the fat you eat, you will probably need to play with the balance of fats in your diet. In the western world, especially in the UK and US, we generally consume a lot of saturated fat. People who live in southern Europe tend to have a better fat balance as they generally eat less dairy, more fish, more plant oils and much more fruit. Think of your favourite region of the Mediterranean and imagine being a local there. How do they eat? French, Italian and Spanish people who live in the countryside tend to eat well-balanced meals prepared from fresh ingredients, avoiding processed foods. If you must drink a lot of milk, try choosing skimmed or half-fat instead of whole milk.

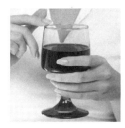
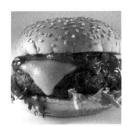

'Except for the vine, there is no plant which bears a fruit of as great importance as the olive.'
PLINY

Defining idea...

39

How did it go?

Q   **If I buy foods marked 'low fat' or 'lite', will I reduce my fat intake?**

A   *If something is low in fat, it may still be high in calories, so you could still be consuming too many calories to lose weight. Compare the label on a low fat product with the standard version of the product.*

Q   **How many grams of fat should we eat a day?**

A   *For average adults of a healthy weight, women should aim for 70 g and men 95 g. When you're trying to lose weight you should be aiming lower. For example, if you are eating around 1800 calories a day, you should go for around 63 g of fat in your diet.*

Q   **I've read about a slimming pill with a fatty acid in it. Does it work?**

A   *Conjugated linoleic acid (CLA) is a fatty acid found naturally in many foods, including dairy products and beef. Back in the early 1990s some researchers found that CLA plays a role in keeping body fat levels low and helping lean muscle tissue to develop. Other studies have since found that CLA can improve the body's muscle-to-fat ratio. A pill containing CLA is not a miracle cure, but there does seem to be enough evidence to give it a try. Remember, though, that you will still have to eat less and increase your level of physical activity. Think of CLA as the icing on the cake, not as an excuse to go back to old bad habits!*

10

Why size matters

It's not just what you eat that counts on the road to losing weight, it's about how much you eat too. How does your sense of portion control measure up?

What do you think a portion size of say, breakfast cereal or meat should be? I hope you're sitting down because it will probably be a shock. I know it is to me every time I see this particular truth in black and white!

According to healthy eating guidelines, a serving of breakfast cereal should be one ounce and a serving of meat should be two to three ounces. Cereal belongs to the food group of which we can have 6–11 servings a day, but it could be very easy to eat all of it at breakfast alone. The meat group, which also includes fish, dry beans, eggs and nuts, should be contributing 2–3 servings a day to our diet. Again, it's astonishing how quickly that can add up.

Here's an idea for you... **Squeeze a lemon. Citrus fruits are a great source of vitamin C and also a phytonutrient called limonoids, which can help to lower cholesterol. These phytonutrients are concentrated in the rind, so try to incorporate the zest of citrus fruits into your cooking. They work especially well in sauces and garnishes.**

The simple fact is that most us eat too much and have lost all idea of what a portion size should be. This is due to a variety of reasons but the most significant is that food is so readily available in our affluent society. We don't have to go and hunt for it – we can just gather it at the supermarket. When eating out or buying takeaways we demand value for money. What better way to appear to offer good value than with enormous portion sizes? At home we'll cook a meal which could serve four or six people, but it's often eaten by just two or four.

Portion control is essential to weight loss. You could be eating all the right things and still gain weight because you're overeating.

Here's a checklist of the sorts of foods we should be eating for a healthy balance of nutrients. It gives a range for the number of daily serving (e.g. 6–11 servings). The upper end of range really intended only for a very active man; most of us, especially sedentary women, should look to the lower end. There are also a few handy little visual ideas of what that amount looks like. It helps to get good at estimating these by eye because you can't carry around a set of scales everywhere you go. Well, you could, but it would look a little obsessive.

...and another **To take your mind off how much smaller your portions may have to be from now on, try a nice swim. It will stop you from eating and thinking about food.**

Bread, cereal, rice and pasta – 6–11 servings

A serving is:
1 slice of bread (the size of an audio cassette tape)
1 small bread roll
2 heaped tablespoons of boiled rice
3 heaped tablespoons of boiled pasta
2 crispbreads
2 egg-sized potatoes
3 tablespoons of dry porridge oats

Swimming burns off some calories, and you can easily turn it into a workout for even more benefits. See IDEA 26, Fancy a calorie-free dip?

Try another idea...

Fruit and vegetables – 2–4 servings of the former, 3–5 servings of the latter

This is based on US recommendations. In the UK, the suggested amount of fruit and vegetables is 'at least 5' a day.

A serving is:

2–3 small pieces of fruit, such as plums
1 heaped tablespoon of dried fruit such as raisins
1 medium-sized piece of fresh fruit such as half of a grapefruit or a melon
1 side salad, the size of a cereal bowl
3 heaped tablespoons of cooked vegetables such as carrots

'A fat person lives shorter, but eats longer.'
STANISLOW LEC, Polish poet and satirist

Defining idea...

Meat, fish, eggs, nuts, dry beans – 2–3 servings a day

A serving is:
60–90 g (2–3 ounces) of cooked lean meat, poultry or fish. This the size of a deck of cards or the palm of your hand.
150 g (5 ounces) of white fish (or three fish fingers)
120 g (4 ounces) of soya, tofu or quorn
5 tablespoons of baked beans
2 tablespoons of nuts and nut products

Milk, yoghurt and cheese – 2–3 servings a day

A serving is:

200 ml milk
1 small pot of yoghurt
90 g (3 ounces) of cottage cheese
30 g (1 ounce) of cheddar or other hard cheese. This is roughly the size of matchbox.

Defining idea...   *'Never eat what you can't lift.'*
MISS PIGGY

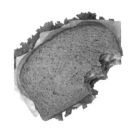
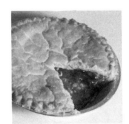

Q   How do you expect me to eat such tiny portions?

How did it go?

A   *Try drinking lots of water. We often mistake thirst for hunger, and most of us don't drink enough water, so this is not just to fill up your stomach. Space out your food by snacking healthily between meals so you never feel ravenous. Don't forget that you can pile up the vegetables – they do fill you up, I promise.*

Q   Are all vegetables equally good?

A   *The majority of vegetables are mostly water (as well as all those lovely vitamins, minerals and fibre), but some are starchy and have more calories. Opt for fewer starchy vegetables and more watery ones. Starchy vegetables include potatoes, peas, corn, squash and turnips. Most of the others, from asparagus to zucchini (courgettes) are watery.*

Q   The only beans I use are tinned baked beans. How can I make good meals out of beans and pulses?

A   *You're not alone! Beans can go into casseroles and chilli sauces, just like meat. Beans and lentils are great in salads and can form the basis for the meal. Ethnic food makes good use of pulses: think of dhal at the Indian restaurant. Tofu, made from soya beans, is often used in Chinese food. There are lots of delicious recipes available. If you're not used to cooking with them, buy ready-cooked beans and pulses in a tin – otherwise you have to cook them for ages and if you don't do it properly you can get an upset stomach.*

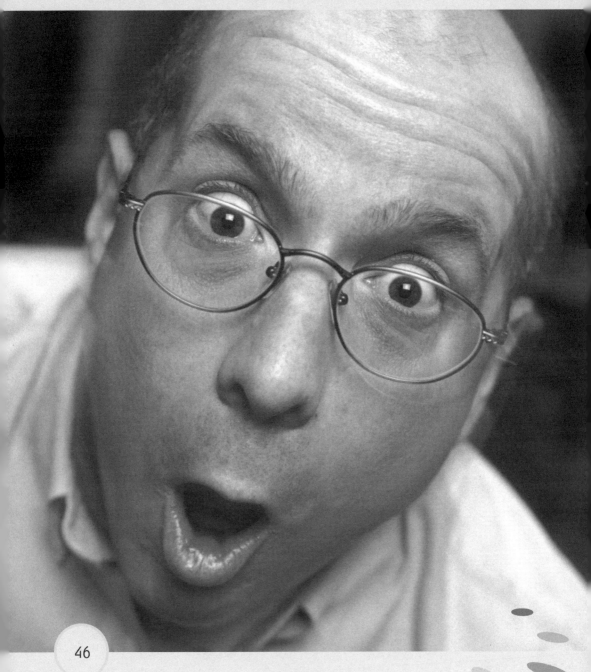

11

With friends like you, who needs enemies?

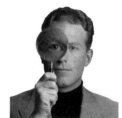

How do you feel about your body? Having a poor body image is a surefire way to sabotage your diet, so shape up with a little self-love.

I know a man who looks like the nerd from central casting. He's overweight, has comedy ginger hair and wears rather thick spectacles, but he truly believes he's a love god.

He really does do rather well with the ladies because he is a fabulous man. He is kind, funny and clever. The point is that he has no problems with his body image. Conversely, in my years as a journalist I have met many of the world's most beautiful women and they have all expressed negative feelings about their bodies, complaining about bellies, cellulite, feeling gawky, ugly and many other 'flaws'. It's not simply a female affliction either – just as many gorgeous men worry about their flabby bellies and 'man breasts'. No one is immune from disliking their shape and looks, but some people seem to manage to get over the problem more readily.

Here's an idea for you... **Dieters often wear black from head to toe because it is 'slimming', but adding touches of colour can really lift your mood. Use red is for energy, blue for communication, green for emotional encounters, yellow for intellectual sharpness and purple when you want to appear calm.**

This is not easy in a society that prizes slimness and makes negative judgements about people who are overweight. It's a prejudice that finds its way into the workplace and relationships, eating right into your self-esteem. The issue intensifies if hating the way you look turns into a negative view of your personality and character. 'I'm fat and stupid' or 'I'm not worth anything, no one likes me' are examples of this kind of dangerous auto-suggestion.

If you don't like yourself, it is going to be really hard to make the lifestyle changes that will help you lose weight. Often these sorts of thoughts are coupled with the habit of comparing yourself with others, especially with images in the media of celebrities and models. The truth is that these people's lives depend on how they look and they have the time and money to spend on an array of products, services and people who will keep them looking fabulous. What's more, the images you see are often 'improved' – for example, photos of models are often airbrushed to remove 'flaws'. For most of us, comparing ourselves to the thin and famous is just going to be a recipe for misery. That's rule number one: don't do it.

You need to develop a more realistic picture of how you would like to look: to look like you, but in better shape. Once you have done that, you can try some other self-esteem boosting tricks. Try writing down all the things you like about yourself, then turning them into positive statements and saying them to yourself every day like a mantra. If that seems too hard, ask your friends or family to write down what they love about you. You never know, you might finish up discovering things you had never even dreamt of that will warm the cockles of your heart.

Next, if someone pays you a compliment, accept it without putting yourself down. Avoid conversations like this:

Friend: 'You look really well.'

You: 'Yes, but I really need to lose some weight because hardly any of my clothes fit anymore.'

Instead, try something like:

'Thanks. I feel great, too. How are you?'

Exercise is good for your self image. Not only will you see physical results, but you'll feel benefits, from the satisfaction of doing something positive for yourself to a greater sense of wellbeing. Exercise has been proven to stave off depression.

Finally, rather than seeing your body as a collection of parts that you think are awful or could use improvement, focus on it as a whole and think of the wonderful things you have done or will do with it. Cuddle someone, run a marathon, give birth, climb trees, build something, help old ladies across the road.... it's your list, you finish it.

Focusing on being a healthy weight is a realistic goal. For more on weight and shape, turn to IDEA 1, *A weighty issue (or, a weighty question).*

Try another idea...

'God made a very obvious choice when he made me voluptuous: why would I go against what he decided for me? My limbs work, so I'm not going to complain about the way my body is shaped.'
DREW BARRYMORE

Defining idea...

How did it go?

Q I'm very self-conscious about my weight and dread meeting new people. What can I do?

A *Meeting new people is daunting for most of us. Studies show that everyone thinks they look worse than they do! The solution is to use the kind of body language that says to others that you're confident and interesting. Rather than avoiding eye contact and slouching away, stand up straight, shake their hand and look them in the eye. If you're sitting at a table try leaning in towards someone: it gives them the signal that you're really interested in what they have to say.*

Q My poor self-image has a knock-on effect to other areas of my life. Sometimes I feel down about everything. How can I change?

A *Try the Wheel of Life exercise, which is one of my favourite life coaching techniques. Draw a circle and divide it into eight segments. Give each of those segments a label that represents an area of your life, such as looks/weight, health, money, work, love and so on. Taking the middle of the circle as 0, or satisfied, and the outer edge as 10, completely dissatisfied, make a cross on each spoke to rank your feelings about each area. When you've finished, join up the crosses. The lowest three scores are the areas you really need to focus on. If you really do feel down more often than up, do go to see your doctor for professional help. There are plenty of things your doctor can suggest, so don't just suffer – make an effort to find a solution.*

12

Why exercise makes you feel on top of the world

You may hate the idea of it, but taking exercise is life-changing and has real benefits for dieters. Once you get into the exercise habit, you won't want to stop.

I think the reason that so many of us are put off formal exercise as adults is a hangover from childhood. I detested Physical Education at school because I was useless at most sports.

At school there was cross country running on a cold winter's morning, followed by a cold shower. As I got older, however, I discovered exercise I liked. For me it was aerobic dance classes in the wake of Jane Fonda's 'feel the burn' trend. I couldn't wait to get into my leotard, leg warmers and head band and leap around like crazy for an hour. That was over twenty years ago and I still go to the gym four or five times a week.

That's the key to incorporating exercise into your life – it has to be something you enjoy. I do believe there's something for everyone. Some of us love swimming. For others, it's running or tennis. These days gyms have a huge variety of classes on

Here's an idea for you... **Keep a log of your TV viewing time over a week. If you watch TV for more than four hours a day, you'll consume more calories than you need to because you'll have more opportunity to snack and you'll burn fewer calories while you are still.**

offer, ranging from the highly choreographed to gentle classes featuring very simple moves. There's no excuse for at least not trying some of them out. If you really don't like gyms, there is walking, which is a very good exercise indeed. It is easy to get into the habit of taking regular walks. Just one foot in front of the other, walk out of your door and keep going.

Why bother to exercise? I'll give you seven compelling reasons:

■ Exercise uses up calories. You will lose weight by cutting down on the calories you consume, but if you're active too, your weight loss will be faster. I love food and working out means I can eat more. It also means that I don't end up losing any weight, but just maintain the weight I am. When you exercise you build up muscle, which gives you shape; even thin people can use muscle tone. Muscle burns up more energy than fat tissue.

■ Exercise gives you a buzz. You've probably heard of the runner's high, that happy, almost euphoric feeling during an exercise session. Experts put it down to a combination of factors – a release of endorphins, hormones that mask pain and produce a feeling of wellbeing; the secretion of neurotransmitters in the brain that control our mood and emotions and a plain old sense of achievement. Whatever gives you the high, there's no doubting the feel-good glow it gives you.

■ Exercise boosts your confidence. Every time you work out or play a sport, you're doing something positive for yourself, which is mood-enhancing in itself. When you start to see the results in the mirror, your self-esteem rockets. As soon as you see results, you will find it easier to stick to your weight loss plan too.

Could a detox diet be a short cut to weight loss? See IDEA 20, *Detox diets – con or cure?*

Try another idea...

- Exercise reduces your appetite. As well as being a good distraction from the allure of the fridge, exercise slows the movement of food through your digestive system, so it takes longer for you to feel hungry.

- Exercise helps you keep weight off. The trouble with only tackling your weight loss from a dietary perspective is that it is usually quite hard to maintain your weight loss in the long term. Once you have reached your goal and are a little less strict with yourself, the weight can begin to come back. Studies have shown that people who have successfully lost weight by taking exercise as well as a sensible approach to food are better at keeping their weight stable long-term.

- Exercise really can be fun. Depending on what you choose to do, you could discover a whole new social circle. I know a few people who met their partners on the Stairmaster at their gym! Don't imagine that everyone else at the gym will be gorgeous. Only the very expensive gyms are stocked with beautiful, thin and rich people – the heaviest weights they lift are their Louis Vuitton bags. Avoid them unless you're looking for someone beautiful, thin and rich.

- According to studies at the New England Research Institute, regular, vigorous exercise can be effective at lowering men's risk of impotence.

'If you think it's hard to meet new people, try picking up the wrong golf ball.'
JACK LEMMON

Defining idea...

How did it go?

Q I am thinking of taking up yoga. Will it help me to lose weight?

A *Yoga and other mind/body exercises involving stretching are wonderful for flexibility and toning. They are also fantastic for teaching you an awareness of your body's strengths and weaknesses and help you to manage stress. They won't do much for your weight loss plan, however. To burn a significant amount of energy you need to do exercise which will get you moving fast, raise your heart rate and make you sweat, such as walking and aerobics classes. Swimming and cycling are good too, but as your body weight is supported, they burn fewer calories – but you may prefer them because this kind of exercise is less stressful on the body. Good, fast sports like basketball, football and rugby are all great alternatives to gym and studio-based workouts, but more sedate activities, such as golf, don't really cut the mustard. If golf is your thing though, don't give it up; any activity is better than nothing, and if you enjoy something you tend to do more of it.*

Q Is housework a way to get fit?

A *Compared with a gym class or running session, housework does not burn a lot of energy. You would need a big house to clean, too! It's not a sport, but housework does count as activity, and some chores count more than others. Ironing, dusting and washing up are light activity, equivalent to walking along slowly at about 4km/hour and don't count towards fitness targets. Window cleaning, vacuuming and mowing the lawn are classed as moderate exercise, equivalent to brisk walking and doubles tennis, and will help to burn up calories faster.*

13

Let's do lunch

If the weight's not shifting, chew on this: your lunch could be making you fat. But a healthy midday meal is easy when you know how.

In a perfect world, we'd all have a leisurely lunch, lovingly prepared by a diet-savvy chef. Afterwards it would be time for a little siesta while someone else cleared up.

In a perfect world we'd all look like Kate Moss and George Clooney and have a few million tucked away in a Swiss bank account too. Back in the real world, whether we're at home, on the move or stuck at our desks at work, we tend either to bolt down something large and fattening that we grabbed at the shop, or we eat standing at the open fridge because we have no time to prepare a meal. Do you ever delay or miss lunch altogether? I do. Then I make up for it with a yummy chocolate bar and fancy coffee to wake me up mid-afternoon, which is very bad news indeed. The trouble with skipping meals is that you get tired and hungry later, and are likely to make unwise snacking choices. By the way, a large coffee with whipped cream tots up to around 500 calories. Learn to love it black or with skimmed milk for the sake of your waistline!

Here's an idea for you... **Make your own sandwiches – it's the only way to be sure what you're eating. Many ready-made sandwiches contain more than 6 g of salt, which is the total intake recommended per day. Reducing our salt intake from the average 10 g we consume to 6 g could prevent thousands of strokes and heart attacks. Salt is also linked to water retention which makes you feel bloated and loads heavier.**

For most of us, a sandwich is often the simplest way to do lunch, but it can contain an astonishing amount of fat and calories. A popular classic is a chicken and salad sandwich – a white bap or roll filled with chicken, mayonnaise, avocado and a lettuce leaf or two. Let's examine each of these elements:

- White bread doesn't fill you up or sustain you as well as brown and can often leave you craving more carbohydrates.

- Mayonnaise really clocks up the calories – 100 g is around 700 calories and 70 g of fat. Even a lighter, reduced calorie version can contain 275 calories and around 25 g of fat.

- Avocado, whilst providing the healthier mono and polyunsaturated fats, plus vitamin E, is a rich source of calories too.

This shows how easy it is to blow the diet without even realising it! Other lunch date baddies include fatty meats, such as sausage and bacon, which are loaded with saturated fats, big wedges of hard cheeses and lashings of butter for the same reason and the rather innocent looking pickle-type relishes which can contain considerable amounts of sugar and salt.

So what does a healthy slimming sandwich look like? It's on brown bread, contains a lean protein-rich filling such as tuna, chicken, ham, brie or cottage cheese and is stuffed full of salad and vegetables for volume, crunch and vitamins. It doesn't contain mayonnaise. In a shop there may be no alternative to mayo, but at home you could try making your own creamy dressing with low-fat yoghurt and chives or other herbs and spices.

If this has got you thinking, turn to IDEA 18, *Rise and dine*, which is all about breakfast. Did you know that people who eat breakfast are generally slimmer than those who skip it?

Try another idea...

It does get boring having a sandwich every day for lunch and perhaps you're not a sandwich person at all. A big salad featuring lots of tomatoes, peppers and other vegetables, plus low fat protein is always a good alternative midday choice. Just watch the dressing. A vinaigrette swimming pool around your salad will pile on the pounds, so a light drizzle is better. Better still, you can substitute it with some lemon juice and herbs for flavour. A baked potato with some low fat protein and salad is great, too – filling, healthy and diet-friendly. Remember to watch out for ready-prepared fillers as they may be heavy on the mayonnaise. Dessert? Fruit wins every time.

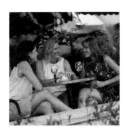

'*Luncheon: as much food as one's hand can hold.*'
SAMUEL JOHNSON

Defining idea...

How did it go?

Q   I eat out for lunch quite often. What should I choose that is light but won't make me look like a diet bore?

A   *Choose grilled meats or fish and steamed dishes, and pile up the vegetables. Opt for tomato-based sauces where possible as they're always less fattening than creamy ones.*

Q   How can I stop the mid-afternoon slump?

A   *Lunches that are high in carbohydrates can make you feel slow by four o'clock. Try balancing your meal with some low-fat protein. The theory is that increasing the protein to carbohydrate ratio will inhibit the release of serotonin in the brain, which, in large amounts, can make you feel sleepy. Try chicken and salad or a ham and salad open sandwich.*

Q   Is it OK if I just drink a large smoothie for my lunch sometimes?

A   *That brings new meaning to the idea of a liquid lunch! It is fine every now and then, but you could get a better nutritional balance by eating proper food. Smoothies can have a high calorie content. I looked at a litre bottle of an orange, mango and banana smoothie recently and saw it contained 600 calories. If you're thinking of a smoothie as a slimming substitute for food, think again.*

14

Are you an emotional eater?

If you find that you often eat without being truly hungry, perhaps it's time to work out what's eating you instead.

On a physical level food is simply fuel for the body, yet our relationship with it is complex. It is a story filled with love and hate.

We read books about food, watch TV programmes about it and pay lots of money to go and eat what someone else cooks for us at restaurants. Over the years we learn habits and behaviours around food that can become inappropriate. These are often rooted in well-meaning parenting. How many of us polish off every last morsel from our plates because mum told us that the poor kids in Africa are starving or that in her generation all they got was bread, potatoes and water? How many of us will have a sweet treat in response to physical or emotional pain, recalling being soothed with confectionary after a childhood fall? We even give foods a moral value – some are bad or sinful, while others are good and virtuous.

Here's an idea for you... **Eat more slowly. It takes 20 minutes for 'I'm full' signals to reach the brain. Work with your body by giving it the time it needs to respond.**

It's a rollercoaster of a relationship, which is fine if you don't have any issues with weight. If you do, and food seems to be controlling you, remember you are not alone. Thousands of us are stuck in this kind of one-way relationship. You need to work out why you are feeding your emotions and what you will do about it.

The desire to eat is masterminded in the brain and involves more than twenty different chemical messengers in your body. Eating anything will stave off hunger, but not overwhelming cravings for a particular type of food. If you are hungry you have to eat, but when you want to eat for any other reason, you need to develop coping strategies that don't involve food. It is usually the negative emotions that drive us to munch more – unhappiness, stress and boredom, for instance. Different approaches work for different people; coping tactics could include talking to a friend, doing some physical exercise, confronting a situation at work that is troubling you or scheduling in some 'me time', such as a fun shopping trip, a facial or a game of golf. The point is to identify the where, when and how of your emotionally reactive eating and deal with that rather than continuing the behaviour that's holding your diet to ransom.

Another trigger can be tiredness. Again, you need to get to the root cause. Are you exhausted because of work pressure or certain relationships? Or is it because night after night you go to bed too late? Tiredness lowers your mood, which makes you want to eat and perk yourself up, and it also makes your body send hunger signals because it is looking for more energy to get you through the day.

My downfall is boredom and procrastination. I often look for the answers to life in the fridge. I can also spend a long time seeking inspiration in a slice of cheesecake, especially the lovely crunchy bit at the bottom. The cure is to do something more interesting than the thing you're putting off. Alternatively, set yourself mini goals; for example, if you finish a task in one hour you will then reward yourself (not with food) before tackling the next task.

Not hungry? Not feeling over-emotional either, yet feeling absolutely desperate for a BLT sandwich? It sound as if you have cravings you need get under control. Flip to IDEA 22, *I want it and I want it now.*

Try another idea...

You don't have to finish up everything on your plate. You could try ordering or cooking a smaller portion to begin with. If you need to assuage guilty feelings, pledge some money to charity for every kilo of weight you lose.

'Stressed spelled backwards is desserts. Coincidence? I don't think so.'
ANONYMOUS

Defining idea...

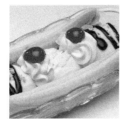
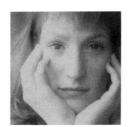
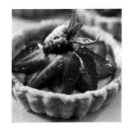

How did it go? **Q I've been trying to consume more good foods since I've been dieting, but I'm not finding them very satisfying. Can you help?**

A *When you say good foods, do you mean those classic diet type foods such as rice cakes, celery, cottage cheese and so on? Have you ever liked those things? If not, don't bother. They are not going to fill you up and make you happy. Go for something you do like, but make it a small portion if it's high in fat. Try buying a low fat/reduced calorie alternative.*

We all tend to perceive some foods as 'good' or 'bad', but I think it is a habit that should be unlearned. Food is just food. Some of it happens to be less calorific or more nutritious. Taking away those sinful/saintly associations gives you a healthier attitude to food, which is the route to weight loss.

Q When I'm unhappy why do I easily devour an entire tub of ice-cream on my own?

A *Fatty foods don't send such strong satiety messages to the brain as carbohydrate or protein-rich foods. A meal with a carbohydrate and protein mix will fill you up for longer, while a high-fat meal or snack will leave you feeling unsatisfied. As a solution to the tub of ice-cream situation, if your diversionary tactics don't work, serve yourself a small portion in a bowl and eat it very slowly.*

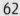

15
Water works

We can't live without water, yet most of us live in a state of dehydration most of the time. Discover the myriad benefits of drinking more water for your diet, energy levels, skin and more.

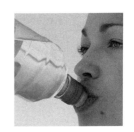

Look through the pages of magazines at the celebrity shots and you'll see that they often carry a bottle of mineral water or have one close by.

It is not because they are being paid a fortune by some water company to endorse their product. They are drinking water because they know it makes their skin glow, look health-conscious and stops them from over-eating. Water is a little miracle. We can't live without it for more than two to five days, but in extremes we can live without food for about a month.

YOUR BASIC BIOLOGY LESSON

Did you know that approximately 60% of an adult's weight is water? Or that two thirds of the water present in the human body is contained within your 50,000

Here's an idea for you... **Buy some softly coloured plates as your crockery could be influencing your appetite. A US study revealed that bold, bright patterns stimulate your hunger, while pastel hues decrease it. Strange, but true.**

billion cells? Water is important. It's not a nutrient in itself, but it is the main component of cells, tissues and blood and is needed for many bodily functions including assisting the absorption of nutrients from food, the regulation of body temperature, the lubrication of our joints and eyes and the elimination of toxins from the body. We lose roughly half a pint of water a day just through breathing.

TELL ME MORE

About a third of daily fluid intake comes from food, not from liquid. Fruit and vegetables generally supply the most water – for instance, salad leaves are mostly water. Our bodies also get water by burning fats and carbohydrates. Experts reckon that we need one and a half litres of fluid a day to stay healthy and more if it's hot or if you're losing extra water through sweating. It is hard to drink too much water, but it is quite easy to not drink enough. Drinking too little water for an extended period can lead to urinary tract infections, kidney and gall stones. You might also find that you suffer headaches, lack energy and have poor concentration. Research suggests that water also plays a role in keeping the skin moisturised and healthy-looking and helps to regulate emotions. So, if you have poor skin and feel cranky and tired, just try drinking more water!

Defining idea...

'It is astounding how quickly skin responds if you drink three pints of water a day. This water cure helps clear impurities from the system feeding the skin.'
HELENA RUBINSTEIN

A feeling of thirst indicates that you are already dehydrated. Thirst is a signal that there is a water deficiency in the cells. Often we interpret this feeling as hunger, so we eat

Going abroad soon? Find your way around foreign menus with IDEA 24, Trip ups.

Try another idea...

rather than drink. This leads quite easily to an unnecessary intake of calories! A large glass or two of water containing zero calories will sort out those 'am I hungry?' feelings. It's important to remember the dehydration spiral: you haven't drunk enough water so you feel hungry and tired, so you snack, but it doesn't make you feel better because you're thirsty, so you eat more before realising you need fluids. Then you feel guilty because you've been snacking, so you snack some more. It's a spiral into more guilt and bad food choices. Break the spiral by drinking frequently, whether or not you think you're thirsty. Eight glasses of water a day is a good target. Take one before and after every meal, and one mid-morning and mid-afternoon.

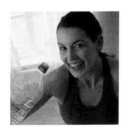

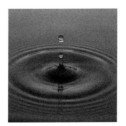

Defining idea...

'*Individuals often find that drinking more water increases the energy levels and can reduce the risk of conditions such as headaches and constipation. However, there is also evidence that a good intake of water is associated with a reduced risk of chronic health conditions.*'
Dr JOHN BRIFFA, quoted on www.naturalmineralwater.org

Q **Does the temperature of the water you drink make a difference?**

A *No. There is a rumour that if you drink iced water, your body needs to work harder to absorb it and hence burns up more calories in the process. Most experts think this is nonsense. Drink it at room temperature, iced or warm – whatever your personal preference.*

Q **Should I drink tap, spring or mineral water?**

A *I think you should drink whatever you think tastes nicest and whatever best suits your pocket. Tap water is perfectly safe to drink, but is subject to treatment so it may have chlorine or fluoride added which you may be able to taste and not be partial to. Spring water comes from an underground source, but may be treated to remove impurities too. Natural mineral water has to come from an identified underground source and be bottled at source, with nothing added or removed except perhaps carbon dioxide to make it fizzy. It must have its mineral analysis on its bottle. Depending on the minerals and their quantity, mineral water may not be suitable for people with kidney problems or for babies to drink. It is fine for everyone else, so if you want to spend the money, feel free to enjoy it.*

16

Metabolism masterclass

Think of your metabolism as your inner energy thermostat. If you turn it up, you will use calories faster, but first you need to understand how it works.

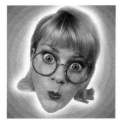

Everyone knows someone who's skinny as a rake and yet could represent their country if eating were an Olympic sport. Meanwhile, a salad seems to go straight to your hips.

We may put this down to having a faster or slower metabolism, but is this really true and if so, can you do anything about it? First you need to get to grips with the science – but there won't be an exam at the end.

Each day your body uses up calories or energy in three main ways. First, there is your basal metabolic rate (BMR), sometimes also known as your resting metabolic rate. This is the number of calories your body would use up if you just lay around all day. The BMR is what your body needs to carry out essential bodily functions, such as keeping your heart beating and breathing. It accounts for 60–75% of your total energy expenditure. *Thermogenesis* is the energy you use to digest food and keep

Here's an idea for you... **For the next week, keep a diary of what and when you eat. Adjusting the frequency of your feeding might give you a boost. Some experts say that eating little and often will boost your metabolic rate because your metabolism is raised by about 10% for a couple of hours after you eat. Others disagree but concede that leaving long gaps between meals can leave you nutritionally deficient.**

warm, which accounts for around 10% of energy expenditure. The last part of the equation is movement, which covers everything from daily activity to sport. This can be from 15 to 30% of energy expenditure.

There are different ways to work out your metabolic rate, which tells you how many calories you use up in an average day. Here's one:

Take your body weight in kilograms (remember 1 kg = 2.2 lb), then, if you are between 18 and 30, multiply your weight by 14.7 and then add 496. This gives you an idea of your BMR. If you are 31–60, multiply your weight by 8.7 and then add 829. With these numbers, think about how active you are. If you take no exercise and mostly sit or stand during the day, multiply your BMR figure above by 1.4. Multiply it by 1.7 if in addition to sitting or standing all day, you also take some exercise, such as brisk walking. If you're very active, moving around a lot during the day and taking regularly exercise, multiply that figure by 2. The final number is the approximate amount of calories you're using each day.

Now back to the BMR. Your genes can play a part in it – some people are born more revved up than others. But you can't change your genes. Your overall body weight makes a difference too. The larger you are, the more calories your body needs for its basic

Are you achieving your weight loss goals? Get on target with IDEA 3, *Setting goals (without always having to move the goalposts)*.

Try another idea...

maintenance. If you lose a dramatic amount of weight very quickly, your BMR will slow, which will ultimately disrupt your long-term efforts at weight control. The best solution lies in building muscle, which burns more calories than fat. Some experts say that an increase in lean body mass can increase energy expenditure by as much as 8–14%. Half a kilo (a pound) of muscle burns 30–50 calories a day, so build 500 g of extra muscle and you'll burn 350 extra calories a week. You can increase your lean muscle mass by weight-training, also known as resistance training or strength training. Anything that puts your muscles under tension counts, so free weights and weight machines in the gym are good, as are choreographed classes which use free weights (usually called something like 'body conditioning'). You could also try a strength-training session at home with an exercise video and dumbbells. One or two sessions a week can really make a difference.

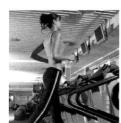 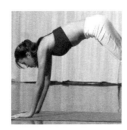

'*Two thirds of people who exercise say it helps reduce stress*'
DR JAMES RIPPE, Center for Clinical and Lifestyle Research, Chicago

Defining idea...

69

How did it go?

Q   Aren't there drugs that raise the metabolism?

A   Yes, but they're not a good idea. Amphetamine-type drugs do speed up the metabolism, but the side effects can be serious – insomnia, depression and anxiety, for example. Herbal supplements can also be risky. Just because something is natural doesn't always means it is safe.

Q   Is it true that yo-yo dieting slows your metabolism?

A   It does in the short term, but recent research has suggested that there isn't evidence that it will have a permanent effect. It is not smart to yo-yo diet, though. Some experts still think that constantly losing and putting weight back on can result in higher overall fat levels. In any case, it does nothing for your confidence and self-esteem.

Q   I have been doing strength training exercise recently and I've put on weight! Why?

A   Have you changed shape? Muscle is three times heavier than fat and takes up less space, so it's possible to shrink in size and weigh more. Rather than keep track of your progress on the scales, try using a tape measure for your chest, waist, hips, thighs and so on. Seeing a difference in cms/inches will be a great motivator.

17

Sweet temptation

Can you refuse the siren call of confectionery? Are you a chocoholic? Here's how to stop a sweet tooth from wrecking your weight loss plan.

Chocolate is like a really great friend. It picks you up when you're down, comforts you, is a pretty good love substitute and would never tell you that your bottom looks really big in your favourite jeans.

The feel-good factor of chocolate and other sweet foods is undeniable. Chocolate does give you a kind of chemical high when you eat it by boosting your brain's serotonin and endorphin levels, making you feel calm and happy. Other substances in it stimulate the brain's emotional arousal, giving you a lovely warm glow similar to being in love.

There's an evolutionary component to the appeal of sweet foods. Human beings have more sweet taste buds than other taste buds and we naturally prefer sweet tastes from babyhood to adulthood. Some scientists believe that humans developed

Try a cup of fennel herbal tea after having a little taste of something you crave. This will suppress your appetite, ensuring you don't carry on munching.

a preference for sweet things because generally they are higher in calories and so pack lots of energy – important in hunter-gatherer times, but less so now that all you have to do is get off the sofa and go to the kitchen cupboard when you feel a bit peckish. If we were as active as we were in hunter-gatherer days and had to work hard to find our food while beating off woolly mammoths, we could stuff our faces with sweet treats and probably wouldn't put on a gram. Times have changed, but we still have our prehistoric tastebuds.

Chocolate is high in fat, often around 30% by weight, and full of calories. Other confectionery is crammed with sugars and can weigh in at 375 calories per 100 g. They will both give you a temporary rise in blood sugar and a feeling of satisfaction, but then your body will tell your brain that it didn't supply all the nutrients it wanted. Your hunger is stimulated and if you continue to munch on the sweet stuff, the process just repeats itself. The high and low swings are in response to your body asking for nutrients, not sugar.

Defining idea...

'*Research tells us that fourteen out of any ten individuals likes chocolate.*'
SANDRA BOYNTON, *Chocolate: The Consuming Passion*

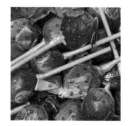

When you're trying to lose weight, it is accepted practice to stay off sweet stuff. In my experience, total denial doesn't work because the more you tell yourself you can't have

Distract your sweet tooth with a different kind of passion. See IDEA 42, *The birds and the bees*

Try another idea...

something, the more you want it. So, here's the deal. Do have a little of what you fancy, but it really does have to be a little portion. Take time to really enjoy it – sit down at the table or on a comfy chair without distractions and savour every mouthful. This way you can make giving in to temptation a positive experience while not over-eating.

You could also try having your sweet hit in a different way. For example, if you want something chocolatey and a bit creamy, make yourself a milkshake using skimmed or non-fat milk and chocolate powder, or have a hot cocoa made half with milk, half with water. A small pot of low-fat chocolate mousse might hit the spot, too. If it is crunch and chewiness you're after, try a thin scraping of chocolate spread on bread, crackers or rice cakes. A meringue with some fruit and a dollop of low fat yoghurt, fromage frais or crème fraiche on top satisfies the need for a pudding without the fat and calorie overload. Get used to reading the labels of your favourite biscuits, cakes and confectionary. By comparing and contrasting, you'll see that some sweet indulgences are much more diet-friendly than others. Life would be so much easier if you just craved broccoli, wouldn't it?

'After eating chocolate you feel god-like, as though you can conquer enemies, lead armies, entice lovers.'
EMILY LUCKETT

Defining idea...

How did it go?

Q **Could I use honey or brown sugar to satisfy my sweet tooth?**

A *Yes, if you prefer their taste, but remember that just because something is not white and granulated, it doesn't mean it isn't sugar. Think about the number of calories you are taking in.*

Q **I've read that chocolate has some useful minerals in it and is good for you. Is this true?**

A *Yes, it contains potassium. Plain chocolate also offers iron and magnesium, but don't forget that these nutrients are coming in a fat and calorie gift-wrapped package. You can get them from other food sources at less cost to your figure.*

Q **Don't you think that if I give in to temptation and just have a bit of something sweet and nice, I won't be able to stop?**

A *You have to stop eating and start doing something else. You could: go for a walk, go to the movies, read a book, go to an evening class, have a cuddle with someone you love, have a long soak in the bath or learn to play a musical instrument. You need to distract yourself and also get absorbed in something that is more interesting (or at least as interesting) as eating.*

18
Rise and dine!

If you thought skipping or skimping on breakfast would be a good way to shed weight, you need to wake up to the fact that the opposite is true. Feast on this.

Wouldn't it be great if there was a really simple trick that made us feel full of energy and sharp as a very sharp thing for hours on end? Well there is, and it is called breakfast.

Many people give breakfast a miss because they think it will help them lose weight. Research has shown that breakfast eaters tend to be slimmer than breakfast skippers. This is due in part to the fact that eating a healthy breakfast keeps you feeling full for longer. That means you'll be more able to resist a quick calorie-laden snack when you're feeling faint at 11 a.m.

Further studies have concluded that if you eat a high carbohydrate breakfast, especially breads and cereals, you'll end up consuming less fat in your daily calorie intake than if you skip breakfast. This is of significance when you're trying to lose weight. Breakfast eaters have been found to have lower cholesterol levels than non-breakfast eaters and those who choose high fat fry-ups.

Here's an idea for you...

Next time you're in the multiplex, think *Amélie* not *Slasher Vixens 2*. Heightened emotions may trigger a desire for comfort food, according to a medical study. Horror films and comedies caused a group of women to eat more, especially the women who had previously voiced concerns over their weight. Travel shows made all the women eat less. Stay calm to lose weight!

Here are a few more good reasons why having breakfast makes sense. According to one UK study, volunteers who consumed a low-fat, high-carbohydrate breakfast reported feeling less tired and muddled than those who ate nothing or chose a high fat, low carbohydrate meal. Studies on school children have shown that kids who breakfast show greater concentration in class, as well as increased problem-solving and verbal fluency abilities. This must also have some application to adults, as has been proven in tests on memory stimulation and breakfast eating. I expect you can guess that adult breakfasters showed superior skills in memory tests than those who went without!

What should you have for breakfast? Fry-ups are out, apart from a once a week treat. But you have to promise to grill your bacon rather than fry it and to choose low-fat sausages. Could you try poaching or scrambling your eggs without adding extra fat? Cereal, whether it is based on wheat, corn, rice, bran or oats, can be a good high-fibre, low fat choice – with skimmed or non-fat milk of course. Do check the label on the packet, as many cereals contain high levels of sugar. Muesli, despite its sandal-wearing, yoghurt-knitting associations, isn't always as healthy as you might think. Many brands contain vast amounts of sugar, not to mention tasty little additions such as chocolate chips. Go for sugar-free varieties. Cooked oats have been around for centuries – the Roman historian Pliny recorded how early Germanic tribes ate porridge. As the starchy oats are digested slowly, so porridge gives a steady release of energy that lasts for hours; it is one of the most satisfying breakfasts you could choose. The soluble fibre in oats also helps to lower cholesterol levels. Prepare it with skimmed milk and it is very healthy and diet-friendly. You could try making it the traditional Scottish way with water, but personally I find that quite disgusting. Wholemeal toast with a scraping of butter and little low-fat protein is a good choice, too. Muffins, croissants and pains au chocolat are not good. Frankly, they are just cake and have no place on the dieter's plate.

Look at diets in a new way and watch the weight fall off. See IDEA 7, *It's never too late to change your mind.*

Try another idea...

Remember, a decent breakfast will make all the difference to your weight-loss plan and could make you a brighter, more cheerful person to be around.

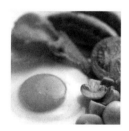
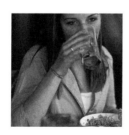

'Eat breakfast like a king, lunch like a prince and dinner like a pauper.'
ADELLE DAVIS

Defining idea...

How did it go?

Q **I really can't face breakfast in the morning. What can I do?**

A *You are not alone, but it is important to try to get into the habit of breakfasting. My suggestion would be that you have something small and healthful as soon as you feel able. A banana smoothie (made with skimmed milk, low-fat yoghurt and fruit) or half a wholemeal roll with reduced-fat cheese are the kinds of foods to go for. Alternatively, just snacking on fruit throughout the morning won't do you any harm, as long as lunch and dinner are well balanced with a mix of low-fat protein and carbohydrates.*

Q **How do I make my own muesli?**

A *All you have to do is soak some oats overnight in some skimmed milk or fruit juice and then add some grated apple, berries or sultanas and a spoonful of low-fat yoghurt or fromage frais. You could also add a handful of nuts or sprinkling of seeds, such as sunflower or pumpkin seeds, which are rich sources of nutrients.*

Q **Is it true that it is good to drink hot water and lemon before eating breakfast?**

A *I don't know of any evidence, apart from anecdotal, that backs up the idea that it will cleanse your system. It won't do any harm and if it makes you feel good, do it.*

19

Walk yourself thinner

If you're new to exercise or just don't fancy the gym, here's a simple way to drop some weight. It's easy to start, and requires no special clothing or equipment.

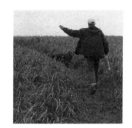

Most of us view walking as a way to get from A to B, and most of the time we'll choose to use the car or bus to get us to where we want to go.

There is a good reason to put one foot in front of the other more often: it's a great way to lose weight and stay slim. It is not expensive, it is not complicated and you can do it anywhere.

Half an hour's walking will burn up an average of about two hundred calories and help to tone up your legs and bottom. There's a catch; you won't see results with a gentle stroll to work or the shops once or twice a week. To make a difference, you'll need to walk at least three times a week, building up to five times a week, for half an hour. You'll need to do it at a reasonable pace, one that warms you up, makes

Here's an idea for you...

Make your dairy product intake low-fat. In research, obese volunteers lost 11% of their body weight over six months on a calorie-controlled diet that included three low-fat dairy portions a day.

you feel ever so slightly sweaty and leaves you feeling slightly breathless, but not so breathless that you could not hold a conversation. If you walk up some hills or on an incline on the treadmill in the gym, you'll increase the challenge and burn up more calories. It is simple. Here are a few other pointers to bear in mind:

■ You don't really need specialist gear for walking, but a decent pair of trainers will support you better than ordinary shoes. If you're planning to take up hill walking or hiking, you will need shoes or boots designed for the purpose, both for comfort and safety.

■ You'll work harder outdoors than inside on a treadmill as you'll have to cope with changing terrain and wind resistance. This is a good thing as you'll burn calories faster and get extra toning benefits. Regularly spending time outside has been shown to keep you emotionally fit too, boosting feelings of well-being and staving off depression.

■ Wear something comfortable! It might sound obvious, but if you get wet or too hot, you'll want to give up and go back home. High-tech sports fabrics are designed to draw away sweat and protect you from wind and rain without weighing you down.

Defining idea...

'Walking is the best possible exercise.'
THOMAS JEFFERSON

■ When walking, keep your tummy muscles pulled in to work your abdominal muscles and protect your back. Walk tall, avoid slumping and use your natural stride.

■ If you swing your arms while you walk, you'll increase your heart rate and get more of a workout.

■ For the best technique, hit the ground with your heel first, roll through your foot and then push off with your toes.

Rather than just randomly walking when you feel like it, try to schedule a daily walk, or at least every other day. That way, you are more likely to stick with it and see results in conjunction with your healthier eating habits, plus you'll be able to monitor your progress.

To reap the greatest benefits, set yourself a plan, say over six weeks, gradually increasing the length of time you walk and its frequency and the speed. For example, in week one you could walk for half an hour three times a week, slowly for 15 minutes and briskly for 15 minutes. Over the next few weeks, you would aim to add another walking session and making each one 5 or 10 minutes longer, and you would walk briskly for 20 or 25 minutes and at a slower pace for the rest of the time. By the end of six weeks, you could be walking for 45 minutes to an hour four or five times a week, and mostly at the faster pace. You'll be seeing a slimmer you in the mirror.

Try another idea...

If you're finding you like the physical and mental effects of exercise, maybe you're ready to challenge yourself further. Go on, I know you want to. Turn to IDEA 21, *Burn fat faster!*

Defining idea...

'A sedentary life is the real sin against the Holy Spirit. Only those thoughts that come by walking have any value.'
FRIEDRICH NIETZSCHE

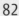

How did it go?

Q   **I love walking, but how do I stop getting lonely?**

A   *Buy or borrow a dog, not just to keep you company, but also to meet other dog-walkers. Could you encourage a friend to come on walks with you, rather than meeting at the wine bar, pub or café? You could also join a walking club, or if there isn't one in your area, set up your own! Although it can be very motivating and help the time pass, for safety's sake I don't recommend listening to music through headphones, especially if you're a woman on your own.*

Q   **Don't you think that walking can get a bit boring after a while?**

A   *There are ways to make it more interesting, like going to picturesque places. This may not be possible every day, but you could drive to a beauty spot for your weekend walking sessions. If you are going to have dinner with friends on the other side of town, why not walk there? You could also sign up for a challenge so that you have a goal to train for. Charity walks can be fun – you meet a lot of people and have the satisfaction of really achieving something, both for yourself and others. There are plenty of organised charity walks at home and abroad, from an easy 5 km walk around your local park to serious trekking in Nepal. Fancy hiking up the Himalayas? Now that's a real challenge!*

20

Detox diets – con or cure?

If you've heard that detoxification diets can help you slim down, you've probably been tempted to try one. But what do they involve and are they safe?

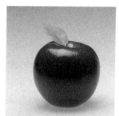

The urge to purge is not a new idea. The ancient Aztecs were keen on enemas, while in 19th-century Europe some doctors argued that removing the colon made sense because it is where the body stores its toxins.

Fasting has long been a feature of some religions. Mostly, however, we're drawn to detoxing as a way to cleanse the body rather than the soul and hope to lose weight in the process. This is what countless magazines, books, celebrities and health gurus sell us.

Detox fans see it as something to be done a couple of times a year to improve digestion, energy levels, skin and to kick-start weight loss. Usually they'll take the pattern of eating only fruit and raw vegetables and drinking juices and water for a few days. Then over the next few days they reintroduce other foods, such as

Here's an idea for you... **Yoga-inspired detox breathing is great for de-stressing and will take your mind off food. Inhale very slowly and deeply, but without straining. Then exhale quickly, as you would if you were sneezing. Continue this breathing pattern and try to become aware of your abdomen tightening and releasing and how calm, heavy and relaxed your body feels.**

steamed vegetables, soups, fish and poultry, wholegrains, nuts and seeds. Red meat, alcohol, coffee and dairy are usually banned. There is nothing wrong with cutting out red meat, alcohol or even coffee, though I have never seen any hard evidence that a cup or two of coffee a day is anything other than delicious.

I don't like the idea of cutting out an entire food group, such as dairy, unless you actually have an allergy. These kinds of detox diets tend to only be for a week or two, and won't do you any harm, but will they do any good? Most doctors agree that your body is perfectly capable of eliminating toxins without the help of a special diet. In fact, the only form of detoxification that many of them recognise is the one for alcoholics when they stop drinking. Believers will counter that the medical establishment is simply behind the times and that because our modern bodies are subjected to pollution and antibiotics and additives in food, they need all the help they can get. Many detox aficionados also claim that the process is cathartic, helping you get in touch with your deepest emotions, which could lead to far-reaching changes in your life. But navel gazing is all you can do when you're light-headed and too weak to get off the sofa. Ouch! That was mean, wasn't it? I do have friends who swear by their January detox and look and feel fantastic. Personally, I find detoxes hard work. I'm for everything in moderation: eating low fat and healthily, with plenty of variety. If you want to avoid pesticides and additives, buy organic food.

FASTING

**Beware of disordered eating.
See IDEA 36,** *Dieting danger.*

*Try
another
idea...*

This is a step beyond detox diets, but is also
recommended as a way to cleanse and boost weight loss. The problem with fasting
is that it makes you feel weak and dizzy, and any weight you lose will find its way
back as soon as you eat normally. The bottom line is that the occasional one-day fast
won't hurt you, but please don't try it for longer than a day unless you're under
professional supervision. Psychologists have commented that fasting attracts
individuals who want to punish their bodies. It's hard not to be down on yourself
when you're overweight, but don't punish yourself. Self-loathing and guilt are
common feelings experienced by dieters, but they sabotage your good intentions
and progress. A healthy attitude to food and your body is the secret of success.

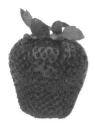
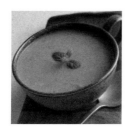

*'I believe this idea of the
build-up of toxins is absolute
rubbish and I won't change
my mind until the detoxing
lobby can prove what they
claim with properly
controlled trials'*
PROFESSOR JOHN GARROW, quoted
in *Zest* magazine

*Defining
idea...*

Q   I think I'd find a full-on detox too difficult. Is there a sort of detox-lite I could follow?

A   *You could try cutting out processed foods, alcohol and sugary products such as cakes, ice-cream and confectionery for a week and see how you get on. You are bound to lose a few kilos. It's really just healthy eating, so it should get you thinking more about the food choices you normally make. It may also stimulate your palate and you could find you prefer the taste of real food to refined foods.*

Q   What about herbal detox drinks?

A   *Readily available in health food stores and chemists, these drinks make the same sorts of cleansing and weight management claims as many other diets. I can honestly say, having tried a few, that I haven't experienced any great effects. One or two have made me feel more energetic than usual but I lost no weight. Try them yourself if you don't mind spending the money. Just don't expect miracles.*

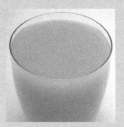 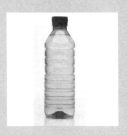

21

Burn fat faster!

Eating less and moving more will result in weight loss. If you rev up the exercise part of the equation, you'll lose kilos quicker.

Taking a bath burns calories. And, given the choice, who wouldn't prefer a nice long soak to a nice long session on the rowing machine in the gym?

Most daily activities, such as watching TV, doing housework and sleeping use energy, but they are unlikely to exceed your energy intake from food. The secret to burning fat faster is to maximise the fat-burning potential of everything you do, from your daily chores and activities to proper workouts. Here are some tips for you to mix and match as you like.

Try working out for longer
If the prospect of an intense workout at the gym or a 15 km hike around your local park horrifies you, try working out less fast, but for longer. For example, walking briskly for an hour burns the same amount of calories as running for half an hour.

Following a good workout, after an hour, go for a healthy protein and carbohydrate snack, such as a tuna and salad sandwich. This will help your body through its 'after-burn', when it replaces short-term energy loss with energy from your fat stores.

Have a more energetic day

You can burn up to 300 calories more simply by being more active in the way you do everyday things. Instead of ambling along to work, stride briskly. Do those dull old household chores you've been putting off for ever, such as cleaning the windows, scrubbing the kitchen floor, tidying the garden and redecorating the bedroom. Put some good old-fashioned elbow grease into it and you've got yourself a workout. Why not start your day in an upbeat mood and dance to a few songs on the radio or on your CD player? And when you next go to the shops, walk instead of driving or taking the bus.

'Consider joining a group or exercising with a friend. Commitments made as part of a group tend to be stronger than those made independently.'
AMERICAN COLLEGE OF SPORTS MEDICINE fitness book

Build some muscle

Use weights, either on gym machines, in a workout class or as part of a home fitness routine. This will help you burn fat and not just because simply lifting weights uses energy. Pumping iron (I know, it's such a male term, but women, please take note) builds muscle tissue, which is metabolically more active that fat tissue. Muscle uses more energy than fat just to exist, so the more muscle you have, the more calories get used, even when you're resting. You really don't need to look like Arnold Schwarzenegger for this to be true.

Learn to love intervals

I don't mean going off mid-performance to have an ice-cream or a glass of wine, I mean interval training. The idea is that you can increase the amount of calories you burn during any exercise by increasing your speed, the intensity or the duration, even for brief intervals. If you are walking, swimming or cycling, you could go steady for about 15–20 minutes, then go faster for a couple of minutes, then slow down again and speed up in random bursts. To earn extra good marks, increase the duration and frequency of the intervals of harder work. It's tough, but really effective.

Remember, the fitter you are, the better your body becomes at using its fuel, which translates into a leaner, more toned you. The more exercise you do, the quicker you'll see results. This makes it worth learning to love exercise.

Weight loss is about calories in versus calories out. But where do they hide and how many do you need anyway? Turn to IDEA 2, *Food accountancy made simple.*

Try another idea...

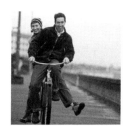
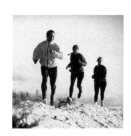

'My idea of exercise is a good brisk sit.'
PHYLLIS DILLER

Defining idea...

How did it go?

Q **I don't really want to pump iron and get lots of muscles. What kind of exercise should I do in the gym that avoids muscle development?**

A *To bulk up you need to use specific training techniques and work very, very hard – much harder than a normal, regular exerciser could ever dream of. Don't give it a second thought, since you won't suddenly become the Incredible Hulk without trying. Instead, think about this: kilo for kilo, muscle takes up less room than fat. This is why many women who take up weight training find they drop a dress size.*

Q **When I lift weights, my muscles go all shaky. What's that about? Is it a sign that I'm ill?**

A *It sounds like it's a normal reaction, and that you are doing good things in the gym. For the best results when weight training, you need to repeat the exercise until you experience muscle exhaustion – that's when you think you really can't squeeze out another repetition and, you guessed it, your muscle starts to shake. If you give up before you reach this point, you're not working hard enough and won't see the results you want. If you've only just started exercising, you might well reach this point after four to five repetitions. As you continue, it will take longer and longer to get there.*

22

I want it and I want it now

Run, hide or play dead and a few other bright ideas to control the food cravings that well up in most of us when we diet.

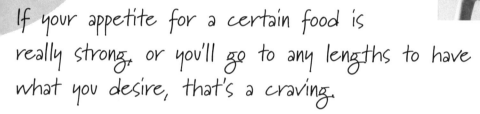

If your appetite for a certain food is really strong, or you'll go to any lengths to have what you desire, that's a craving.

In the past, it has been thought that cravings represent a nutritional need. Some experts, especially those with an alternative medicine background, still maintain that is the case. I think it's rather curious that we invariably crave sweet, fatty things as opposed to a nice big serving of spinach. There is no doubt that at certain times your cravings can be related to what is going on in your body. This seems to be particularly true for women and may be hormone-related. Many women experience strong cravings just before menstruation, for example. It is also common to have cravings when you're pregnant. I couldn't eat enough baked beans when I was pregnant, which was not very glamorous. Men don't get so many cravings. It seems we all grow out of cravings in the end; the over-65s have fewer cravings than younger people. It is thought this is because our appetites reduce with age, together with a weakening of the senses of smell and taste.

Green tea can raise the metabolic rate. If you drink four or five cups a day, you could burn up around 70 calories – for doing very little! Drinking green tea could lose you nearly half a stone over a year. Put the kettle on!

The bad news is that people who are trying to lose weight experience the most cravings. Much of this can be put down to psychological factors. Remember when, as a child, you were told not to do something and it made you want to do it even more? It's the same with dieting. Self-denial in itself just makes you want to have whatever you have told yourself you are not allowed to have.

Diets that are very restrictive become incredibly dull and foods that are banned become disproportionately attractive. In contrast, a healthy long-term approach to losing weight, using a balance of nutrients and portion control, won't encourage cravings because there's no real deprivation. You also won't become desperately hungry if you're eating sensibly, which will curb cravings and mean that the double cheeseburger and fries you are fantasising about will remain in the burger shop where they belong.

If a craving sneaks up on you like an uninvited guest who won't take the hint that you don't want their company right now, you could try one of these three tricks:

■ Bring on a substitute.

  If it's chocolate you're craving, would a glass of chocolate milk made with skimmed milk do? You could try grating a couple of squares of chocolate on top. If the subject of your lust is ice-cream, go for a lower fat version or try sorbet.

■ Pay attention to portion size

Buy a smaller version of your favourite food craving, such as a kid's size, a travel size, just not a family size! This way you can't overindulge. Or, measure out a small portion of what you fancy, sit down and really concentrate on enjoying it. When you've finished, get involved in a non-food related activity.

■ Give in and don't beat yourself up

Denying yourself a craving could lead to a full-scale binge.

It's also worth seeing if you can identify a pattern in your cravings – for instance, check if they occur at certain times of the day. Work out if how you usually feel at that time of the day. The more you understand your eating habits, the easier it is to tackle them and not allow them to interfere with your goal to lose weight.

Exercise helps to control your appetite. If you're not a gym fan, read IDEA 35, *Shape up from home*, which suggests another approach,

Try another idea...

'Food is like sex. When you abstain, even the worst stuff begins to look good.'
BETH McCOLLISTER

Defining idea...

93

How did it go?

Q   Why is my craving for sweet foods intensified when I'm premenstrual?

A   *Lots of women say that they experience this. Our bodies do require extra calories just before menstruation. The trick is to improve the overall balance of your diet. You could also try taking a multivitamin supplement with zinc and evening primrose oil. Don't deny yourself, but be careful not to binge. As well as employing distractions, this is also a time of the month when you could probably use some pampering. A massage, for example, will make you feel good, and lessen the bloated, cranky feelings of PMS. It will also stop you thinking about food for a while.*

Q   Are there any ways I could 'train' myself out of a craving, like you train a puppy not to do certain things?

A   *You could try 'de-temptation' training. List six or seven foods that you regularly crave and put them in order of importance. Take the food craving you care least about from your selection and carry some of it around with you all day in your bag, briefcase or pocket. At the end of the day throw it away or give it to someone else. Work through your whole list to prove to yourself that you can resist giving in to your cravings. Some people swear by this method, and even if it doesn't completely remove the cravings, you'll probably learn quite a lot about the whys, whens and hows of these unwelcome urges.*

23

Make your kitchen more diet-friendly

Decent equipment and a little low fat cooking know-how can transform the way you eat. It's fun to learn, too.

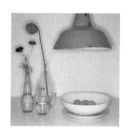

I have heard it said that you should never trust a skinny chef; I never trust them with the double cream, because they just don't care about calories.

The proliferation of celebrity chefs with their TV shows and books is undoubtedly a good thing in as it has definitely reawakened our collective interest in food and cooking. However, these people, pleasant as I'm sure they are, do not care about your diet. What you do in your own kitchen is of paramount importance in the battle of the bulge. The good news is that it's easy to serve up food that is calorie-conscious, yet still delicious. Here, in no particular order, are a few of my top tips for slimmingly wonderful food preparation methods and techniques:

1. Get used to grilling as a less fattening way to cook meat and fish than frying. You can do it without using any extra fat at all. If you find that your grilling is getting a bit dry, simply brush on a small amount of an unsaturated fat, such as olive or sunflower oil. Note the word brush; it's quite different to drench.

Here's an idea for you...

Slouching and eating don't mix! Lying down makes you eat more than when you're sitting up straight at a table. When you're lying down, food passes through your gut more slowly and it takes you longer to realise that you are full.

2. Invest in a steamer to cook your vegetables. Boiling boils most of the nutrients away and makes them all school-dinner soggy. You can even be adventurous and steam fish.

3. When serving vegetables, don't dollop a knob of butter on top. A few chopped herbs, such as parsley or mint, add oodles of flavour without the calories.

4. Buy good quality, non-stick cookware so you can reduce or cut out the need for cooking with fat. Nothing lasts forever, though, and non-stick coating can wear off over the years. Check your pans to see if they need replacing.

5. Use proper measures. While it's fun and terribly TV chef to measure using your eye and just throw everything together, in real life this means it is easy to add unnecessary calories and produce overly large portion sizes.

6. Braising and poaching are a couple of failsafe healthy cooking methods that you can use for fish and meat. Just use stock, milk, water or juice and chuck in the relevant herbs and spices.

7. If you're making a casserole or meaty sauce such as Bolognese, you could try dry frying the meat first and draining away the excess fat before you add in your other ingredients.

8. Always look to see if there is a reduced fat version of your ingredients. For example, coconut milk is a staple of many cuisines, but is very high in saturated fat. You can find brands with half the fat, which is worth it if you use it a lot. Double-check that you can use reduced and low fat butter/margarine products for cooking, as some are only suitable for spreading.

What's a healthy balance of foods on your plate? See IDEA 4, Pyramid selling.

Try another idea...

Just because you're losing weight, it doesn't mean it's all bland deprivation in the kitchen department. And if what you are producing tastes like cardboard, add a new cookbook to your shopping list.

'The kitchen is the great laboratory of the household and much of the weal and woe as regards bodily health depends on the nature of the preparations concocted within its walls.'
MRS BEETON, *The Book of Household Management*

Defining idea...

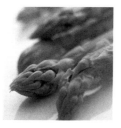 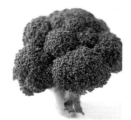

How did
it go?

Q   How can a dish have a creamy texture without cream?

A   *Just add a little reduced-fat crème fraiche or yoghurt. Although it's not the lowest fat option, a light Greek yoghurt has a creamier taste than regular low-fat yoghurt.*

Q   I love bacon and want to cut it out completely, but what substitutions could I make?

A   *In cooking, you could try swapping bacon for sun-dried tomatoes. Rinse the oil off them or reconstitute dry ones in water. They will produce a flavour that is as rich as bacon. You could also try turkey rashers, which look like bacon. They are perfectly tasty and a lot less fatty.*

Q   What about microwaving?

A   *Some people are mistrustful of microwave ovens, but I think they're great because you rarely need to add fat to whatever you're cooking in them. They're also brilliant when you're late, tired or lazy because you can whip up something healthy and tasty in half the time that it would take to go to the take-away on the corner. Make the microwave your friend, and use it to make a wholesome, hot meal instead of giving in to the attractions of commercially prepared take-aways that are full of fat, salt and sugar.*

24

Trip ups

They say travel broadens your mind, but it can also thicken your waistline. Here's how to holiday without piling on the pounds.

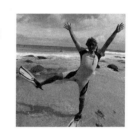

Looking at your holiday snaps can be a turning point in deciding to lose weight. Seeing how plump you look in them can be quite a shock.

I remember eagerly shuffling through my photographs after returning from a sojourn in Portugal. I was looking for the ones in which I might look as though I was related to Cindy Crawford, but no, I looked hideously out of shape from every angle in every picture. There were a lot of me at tables, laden with the remnants of blow-out meals and several empty wine bottles. Cruelly confronted with my personal excess baggage, I vowed that I was going to get a grip and be slim and toned by my next break.

The aftermath of a holiday can be scary, but often it's the prospect of going on holiday that fills us with fear. Away from our normal routines, we worry about how we're going to eat in a calorie-conscious way to avoid returning with an extra three kilos as a souvenir. If you go to somewhere really remote and exotic, you might

Here's an idea for you...

Eat fiddly food. It could save you calories. Things like fresh artichoke, crabs, lobster, shrimps with their shells on, and mussels require some effort to consume, so you eat more slowly. This stops you eating too much too fast.

come home a stone lighter thanks to some nasty tummy bug, but otherwise, travelling and staying abroad is likely to trip up your diet plans.

This doesn't mean that you shouldn't go on holiday! You can't put life, fun and new experiences on hold while you try to get to your target weight. The key is knowing your way around foreign menus, choosing dishes wisely, watching the portion sizes and going easy on the local beers, cocktails, vino, sangria and port or whatever other alcoholic temptations are on offer.

Here's a whistlestop tour of popular holiday destinations and the pros and cons of local cuisine:

SPAIN

Go for: gazpacho, stuffed peppers, grilled fish, salads, paella, mussels, grilled chicken and rice, tortilla.

Skip: fried dishes, whitebait (they're cooked in batter, so it's a snack with more than 300 calories), fish served with oily sauces, albondigas (fatty meatballs) and chorizo (a high fat sausage).

GREECE

Go for: pitta bread, salads, baked fish, stuffed tomatoes, grilled fish, fresh fruit, seafood kebabs, lamb and pepper kebabs, tzatziki and hummus dips. When you order salad, ask for the dressing on the side.

Skip: baklava sweets, moussaka (a high-fat dish), meatballs, taramasalata (just a tablespoon is 50% fat and contains 200 calories), and spicy sausages.

ITALY

Go for: fish dishes, thin-base pizzas with vegetable toppings, pasta with tomato, vegetable or seafood sauces, parma ham with melon, seafood salad, bread sticks, tuna and bean salad, and grilled chicken (ask for sauce on the side).

Skip: pasta with creamy or buttery sauces, pizza with salami, extra Parmesan, chargrilled vegetables (drenched in oil), pesto sauce. Avoid creamy sauces such as carbonara.

FRANCE

Go for: consommé soup, grilled trout, ratatouille, salads, bouillabaisse, salad-filled baguettes, lower fat cheeses such as brie, camembert and goat's cheese, and French onion soup (but don't eat the floating cheese).

Did you know that sleep plays a part in weight loss? Flip to **IDEA 29**, *Snooze and lose*, to find out more.

Try another idea...

'*The trouble with Italian food is that five to six days later you're hungry again.*'
GEORGE MILLER, British writer

Defining idea...

'The quality of food is in inverse proportion to a dining room's altitude, especially atop bank and hotel buildings – airplanes are an extreme example.'
BRYAN MILLER, *New York Times* restaurant critic

Skip: Creamy and buttery sauces such as Béarnaise or à la Normandie, buttered vegetables, patisserie, croissants, and pain au chocolat.

USA

Go for: Tex mex – bean burritos, chicken fajitas, vegetable chilli tostadas, low-fat or fat-free muffins, yoghurts and ice-cream. In the USA you can get any variation on a menu, but you need to ask. The downside is the enormous portions they give you.

Skip: burgers, fries, cheesecake, brownies, potato skins, tortilla chips, fried steaks and Caesar salad, which seems healthy, but has a dressing that whacks up the fat and calories.

THAILAND

Go for: fish cakes, prawn or green papaya salad, stir-fried vegetable dishes, soups (avoid those with coconut, a rich source of saturated fat), meat or seafood pad ka pau (stir-fried with garlic, basil and chilli), whole baked fish.

Skip: Curries (often swimming in coconut milk) and satay sauce (delicious, but a calorie colossus).

Q **I enjoy exercise and want to keep it up while I'm away. Any suggestions?**

How did it go?

A *Ring in advance to check if your hotel has a gym or an arrangement with a local health club. Perhaps they could also assist you in hiring a bike during your stay. You could check if your room has a video so you could take along a couple of exercise tapes. A skipping rope is a fun way to do some cardiovascular work, while a resistance band can take the place of weights. Don't underestimate the benefits of swimming or walking on beaches and around the sights either.*

Q **Although I can control what I eat when I get there, I find the actual travelling tricky. How do I stop eating something that I don't really want because I am too hungry to resist.**

A *The simplest thing to do is to pack your own little food bag for your journey with plenty of fruit and low-fat snacks. That way you won't be caught out and have to eat a burger because there was no choice on the train/at the airport. Don't forget that most airlines can provide for a special diet, as long as they have enough notice. Some are better than others, but it's always worth asking for a low-fat meal or a vegetarian option, which should at least guarantee some fresh fruit and vegetables.*

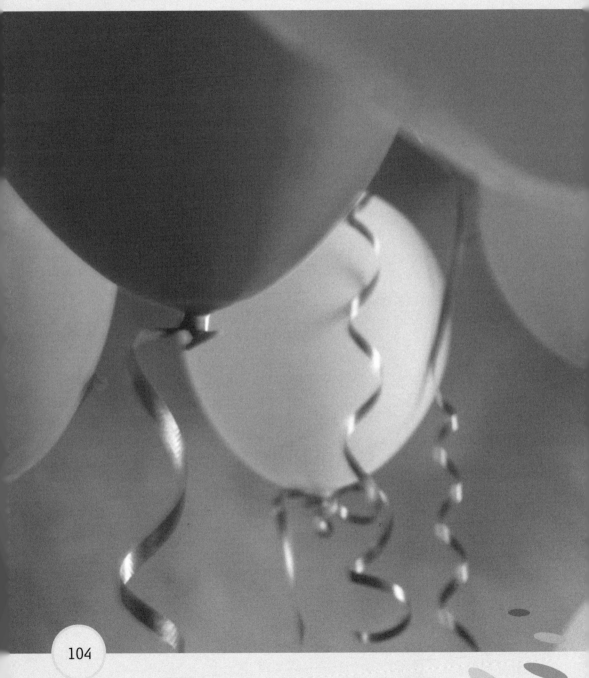

25

The morning after the night before

Special events always seem to be popping up to put your eating plans under severe strain. Here are some tricks to help you stop falling off the diet wagon.

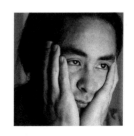

Weddings, birthdays, anniversaries, new job, new home — they are all great excuses for a party and could lead you into temptation. Don't let your good diet intentions fall by the wayside.

It's hard to resist free-flowing alcohol and high-calorie snacks and treats in a happy, loud atmosphere. How easily those handfuls of peanuts can slip down. More wine? How about a cocktail? Have a slice of cake. Taste this cheese. The next thing you know, you've completely overdone it.

Come the morning, you wake up feeling bloated, perhaps a little hungover, cross and disappointed in yourself. Your reaction could be to give up your diet. Or obsess about the precise amount of calories and fat consumed. It's important not to let these negative feelings take over. Firstly, it's unlikely that your one-off excesses will

Here's an idea for you...

Play with plate size. If you eat from an enormous plate, chances are you'll fill it with an enormous portion or feel short-changed because there doesn't appear to be much on it! Choosing a smaller plate and piling it up is a sneaky way to trick yourself that you're having a big meal.

lead to weight gain. You need to overeat by around 3500 calories to put on half a kilo (a pound) of fat. Any bloated, fat feeling you may be experiencing is more likely to be water retention after eating lots of salty foods, such as crisps, nuts, pies, pizza and so on. Take some time to think about how you feel and then reframe your thoughts in a positive way. So for example, instead of dwelling on the idea that as a result of your over indulgence you've totally blown your diet and may as well give up, say to yourself 'I've been losing weight steadily and after my break yesterday, I'm confident and eager to get back to my healthy habits today'. And rather than thinking you can never go to another party because you'll pig out, try to get some learning from the experience. Which foods in particular couldn't you get enough of? Was it the alcohol that was your downfall, both in terms of the empty calories and the fact that alcohol relaxes the willpower? Did you continue to eat when you felt full? Identifying the pitfalls should mean that come the next party, you'll have some tactics to cope. For instance, if you have a soup or salad or piece of fruit before you go out, you'll feel a little fuller and therefore more able to avoid picking at calorie laden-snacks. You could also try having a large glass of water in between every alcoholic drink. Maybe you could mingle with fellow guests in an area away from the food, to avoid

Defining idea...

'One more drink and I'd have been under the host.'
DOROTHY PARKER

snacking without really thinking about what you're doing. Conversation could be another diversionary tactic. After all, it's rude to speak with your mouth full!

As for feeling tired the morning after the night before, you need some damage-limitation tricks. Chances are you'll be craving carbohydrates to boost your energy levels and, if you're hungover, fatty foods too. A healthy eating plan will get you back on track though.

For many of us, losing weight gets harder as you get older. For some good reasons why, immerse yourself in IDEA 33, *Stop the middle-age spread!*

Try another idea...

Start the day with a large glass of water to combat dehydration, then have a slow-energy release breakfast to ensure you don't get snacking urges mid-morning. Try something like porridge, a slice of wholemeal toast, with a thin scraping of butter or low fat spread and jam or reduced sugar baked beans or a smoothie (just blend half a pint of skimmed milk with a pot of low fat yoghurt and some fruit of your choice). Drink another couple of glasses of water during the morning and if you need to snack, eat fruit, crackers and jam, a fruit scone or a rice cake, spread thinly with peanut butter. A huge salad with some low fat protein for lunch should fill you up healthily. If you include watercress in your salad, you could help combat the bloat as it's a natural diuretic. Have an early evening meal of simple grilled fish or meat with plenty of vegetables. If you cut out starchy foods, such as pasta, rice and potatoes with this meal, you'll save on calories, helping to balance out yesterday's splurge. An early night will ensure you look and fabulous the following day!

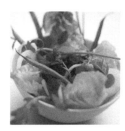

'When I read about the evils of drinking, I gave up reading.'
HENNY YOUNGMAN

Defining idea...

Q **I can't help but mooch around the day after a pig-out. How can I start the day more positively?**

A *Go for a walk, swinging your arms and breathing deeply. You'll feel energised and have burned a few calories. On your walk think about how you'd like to feel today. Keep that feeling in mind and plan how else you could fuel it. Once you get home, rather than slobbing around in an old tracksuit, get dressed up to give yourself a lift. If you need more encouragement, phone a friend or a member your family who you know will make you feel good and who you can have a laugh with.*

Q **It's the buffets that I find the killer at parties. How can I negotiate my way round one in the most calorie-conscious way possible?**

A *Buffets are difficult, especially as it's easy to go back and forth without anyone noticing. Rather than having a little portion, so you feel it's OK to keep going back for more, promise yourself you will make only one visit and put your whole meal on the plate so you can see exactly how much you're eating. Foods to load up with are vegetables and salads. You should also try to stick with lean meats and grilled foods (but check they're not swimming in a pool of oil). Avoid pastry, creamy dips and too many salty snacks.*

26

Fancy a calorie-free dip?

It's easy to turn a dip into a workout. What's more, splashing around is so much fun that it won't even feel like exercise.

Like it or not, we all know that a sedentary lifestyle does us no favours in terms of health and fitness, not to mention the slimming stakes.

Many people shy away from 'formal' exercise such as sports and the gym because they find it dull, hard to do or hard to fit into their lives. That's why I'm suggesting swimming, which most of us view as an enjoyable thing to do rather than a chore. In my experience, there seem to be very few people who really hate it. I am one of those people, but that's because I nearly drowned as a kid and wouldn't go back into to the water for years – so I choose the gym over the pool every time.

Swimming is great exercise, easy on your joints and lots of fun. You can even take your kids along. Just make sure that someone keeps an eye on them whilst you do a little more than splash about, using the following ideas.

Here's an
idea for
you...

Saddle up! Horse riding is a
great alternative exercise
routine. Just sitting in the
saddle strengthens your
stomach and back muscles, and
tones your thighs, bottom and
legs. It provides an aerobic
workout too.

■ **Use different strokes to maximise the
benefits** – If you vary the strokes you use,
you won't get bored with endless laps of
front crawl. Breaststroke works on the chest
muscles, shoulders, upper back, arms and
thighs, while backstroke focuses on the
upper back as well as the arms and stomach
muscles. Crawl works the shoulders and
upper back, the buttock muscles and the
quads at the front of the thighs.

■ **Try floats for extra resistance** – Use a float for extra muscle toning. For the
lower body, simply hold your float out in front of you and kick your legs to work
your legs and bottom. If you hold the float between your legs so you can't kick
them, you can concentrate on working on your arms.

■ **Maximise fat burning potential** – Rather than swimming along at a gentle
pace without getting your face wet, you'll have to get your heart rate up to burn
lots of calories. One way to do this is with interval training, which means
swimming fast for a length or two, then swimming more slowly. Just as you feel
you're starting to recover, pick the pace up again and so on until the end of your
session.

Defining
idea...

'*The cure for anything is salt
water – sweat, tears or the
sea.*'
ISAK DINESEN

■ **Keep it up!** – As with any exercise you have to do it consistently to see results. Swim three times a week for twenty minutes as a starting point and you'll feel fitter and more toned in a month. If you're very overweight, you'll see a difference much sooner. In order to keep seeing results, you should increase the length of time you spend in the pool, and aim for five sessions a week.

> **You've improved your swimming technique, now polish up your shopping skills with IDEA 37, *How to be a smart (slim) shopper.***

Try another idea...

■ **Breathe right** – Breathing correctly stops you becoming exhausted too quickly or getting frustrated at taking in mouthfuls of water. Think of breathing for swimming in the same way as breathing when you're walking down the street. You should neither hold your breath or take in enormous gulps of air. With the crawl, for example, when you need to take a breath just turn your mouth to your right or left shoulder. When you put your head back into the water, look forward rather than down. This will help with exhalation as your windpipe is more open. Breathe out by letting the air trickle out slowly instead of blowing it out. Develop a rhythm and you'll be able to keep going for longer.

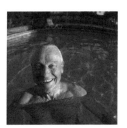

> **Efficient swimmers seem to "knife" through the water with little effort. Like human torpedoes, they streamline themselves to become as small as possible in the direction they intend to move.**
> WES HOBSON, CLARK CAMPBELL and MIKE VICKERS, *Swim, Bike, Run*

Defining idea...

Q **My swimming technique is not really that good – it's limited to back and breast stroke. Am I really exercising properly?**

A *Swimming lessons aren't just for kids. Most pools offer the services of an instructor, so go for it. You'll feel a difference in just a few sessions.*

Q **I want to swim at lunchtime, but by then I'm starving. You can't swim on a full stomach, so what should I do?**

A *Try a quick snack, such as a piece of fruit and a large glass of water, half an hour before swimming. It should take the edge off your hunger.*

Q **I like water, but I get bored with swimming. What can I do to make it more fun?**

A *Try aqua aerobics, which is fun for just about everyone. Some exercises are done holding on to the side and others use floats. Most sessions include some sort of routine in the middle but you're never out of your depth. Try a few different classes, as instructors have different styles, and you'll like some more than others.*

Can beauty products help you slim?

Lotions, potions and treatments promise all kinds of miracles, including inch loss and wobble firming. But are they worth the money?

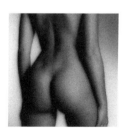

It's an appealing idea. Rub in this cream twice a day for six weeks and your flab will melt away.

A friend of mine once remarked that these creams should come with a symbol on them, featuring a slice of cake with a cross through it meaning that to lose weight, you have to watch what you eat as well as, or even rather than, spend money on some gimmicky product. But he's a cynic and a man – and men generally don't believe in the powers of applying creams to themselves. They prefer it if you do it for them, coupled with a back rub, after eating a fabulous meal you've cooked for them, and that you've also shopped for and cleaned up after – not to mention put the kids to bed, fed the cat and done a little recreational vacuuming. But enough man-bashing. This idea is as much for them as it is for women.

Here's an
idea for
you...
Get a fake tan. It can make you look slimmer and leaner by sculpting, shadowing and highlighting muscles and curves. For the best results, have it applied in a salon. It will usually last for about five days.

Depending on your background, beauty treatments can be very useful for getting in shape or a waste of time, money and effort. The cosmetics industry is always able to wheel out a boffin from their laboratories to produce clinical studies proving that X cream really does help you lose inches, refine your silhouette or firm your curves. Meanwhile, most other doctors and scientists will say that what you apply from the outside doesn't make a blind bit of difference. Advertising claims are strictly regulated and can only go so far, so it can be hard to know how effective these products really are. The better magazines and newspapers do some investigatory work and produce information and recommendations of their own.

I believe that some of these treatments do have an effect, though it might be short-lived. I also think that the psychological element can't be underestimated. There's no doubt that looking after yourself does make you feel good. When you feel good, you're motivated, positive and confident, which is how you need to feel to spur you on to losing weight.

Here are my opinions of what's on offer:

SALON TREATMENTS

These usually involve being wrapped, massaged or painlessly zapped with some sort of electrical current. Massage is undoubtedly soothing and is claimed to stimulate your lymphatic system, which drains waste fluid from your tissues. You'll feel good afterwards, but not thinner. Wraps can shrink inches, but it's just fluid loss – they are fab for feeling a bit thinner for a special occasion. You can't beat them for a short-term boost. Electrical impulses stimulate your muscles by working them while you lie back and read a magazine. You would see better results with regular exercise.

For more on looking good while you're going down in size, see IDEA 38, *Alternatives to kaftans.*

Try another idea...

FAT-BUSTING CREAMS

Despite the claims, I really don't believe you get results unless you eat less and move more too. Still, they do make your skin feel very smooth and soft and strokable.

COLONIC IRRIGATION

This is very controversial. It is based on the principle that toxic deposits are stored in your large intestine. When these are flushed out, it kickstarts the metabolism and helps elimination. If having a speculum inserted in your anus and having gallons of water sloshing around your insides is your idea of a good time, go right ahead! While many alternative practitioners say it's perfectly safe and even emotionally rewarding, conventional doctors reject the idea, even saying it's downright dangerous.

'After forty a woman has to choose between losing her figure or her face. My advice is to keep your face and stay sitting down.'
BARBARA CARTLAND

Defining idea...

115

How did it go?

Q **A friend recommended skin brushing as a way to combat cellulite. Will it work?**

A *I am a fan of skin brushing. This is where you stroke a dry bristle brush in sweeping movements over your limbs and torso, always working towards the heart. It definitely makes your skin feel great and gets the circulation going. I don't think it will get rid of cellulite, though used in combination with massage, diet and exercise, it will help to hold it at bay.*

Q **I read about some slimming tights recently. Can you tell me more?**

A *Coffee tights look like normal tights but are impregnated with caffeine which slowly gets absorbed through the skin. The idea is that this speeds up the metabolism, leading to inch loss. One test had all the volunteers losing inches from their waists and hips. Usually I'd be cynical, but I think I might just give these a go myself. You can find out more at www.palmers-shop.com.*

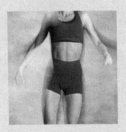 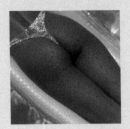

28

Members only

Slimming clubs promise results, but who are they for and will they make more of a dent in your pocket than your fat reserves?

Our reasons for finding it easy to gain weight and hard to lose it are as individual as our musical preferences. If yours include a lack of motivation and encouragement, try a slimming club.

Millions of people the world over belong to slimming organisations. Although the majority of clubbers are female, men are signing up too. Experts agree that the big established clubs do a good job, by providing support, which is incredibly important when you're trying to lose weight. They also offer plenty of information, advice and tips on long-term weight loss. Of course, not all clubs are created equal; for example, some are more expensive than others. Some include an exercise session, while others barely mention exercise at all. Before joining up, it's a good idea to prepare a list of questions that you can ask the trainer or group leader. This way you should be able to work out if the club will be right for you. Try these for starters:

Get everyone in your office or household to write down their favourite comfort foods. Notice any gender bias here? Men and women eat different kinds of comfort food. Men prefer things like mashed potato and pasta, while women prefer instant snacks such as chocolate and biscuits. Is this because men don't expect to have to cook them for themselves?

1. Is there any evidence that this club's methods work? As well as testimonials and member success stories, do they have any press clippings from magazines and newspapers? Are these publications independent, or do they only have clippings from their own in-house publications?

2. What are the costs and payment structure? Will you have to pay extra for special sessions, special foods or supplements recommended by the club?

3. How convenient will the meetings be for you, both in terms of time and geography. Are there options to follow the programme on–line or by post?

4. What are the club rules? Does it focus solely on diet, and if so, what are the basic guidelines you will follow? Is exercise included in sessions or recommended? Do they have vegetarian options? Ask about things like motivational talks and image consultants – these are extras that will really give you value for money.

Defining idea... *'I have a mind to join a club and beat you over the head with it.'*
GROUCHO MARX

5. What would a typical day's menu look like? Better to find out now!

6. What about aftercare? When you reach your target weight, do they offer a maintenance plan? Is that included in the price, or does it cost extra?

7. Can you sit in on a session to see what it's like? Getting a feel for the format, what's expected and what the other members are like, is so important – make sure you feel happy with the support network on offer.

Have you discovered the wonders of water yet? It's great for your energy levels, for your skin and, of course, your waistline. Go to IDEA 15, *Water works*.

Try another idea...

As well as the big name diet clubs, your local doctor or hospital may well run a weight-loss programme, and your local gym may offer one too. Do not respond to flyers, posters and funny little ads in newspapers saying something like 'Wanted! Overweight people to lose 30 lb in 30 days. No hunger! No Exercise!' These sorts of operations usually have a product they are pushing hard, such as a slimming pill or a meal-replacement shake. You may well be invited along to a meeting where various 'before and after' case studies will be trotted out in front of you and a few salespeople will speak with evangelical fervour about the product. Then, *bam!* 'Here's your month's supply.' And have you guessed? It costs nearly as much as your monthly salary. Seductive as it might seem, losing a vast amount of weight quickly is not sustainable. It will be water and lean muscle mass that disappears, only to reappear when you start to live normally again. If you try to do it with some unproven diet pill you could be putting yourself in all kinds of other health dangers, too. Go for the tried and tested methods.

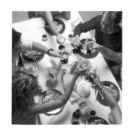

'*Women are more likely to lose weight and keep it off in a group than on their own.*'
BBC Diet Trials 2003 findings

Defining idea...

How did it go? **Q   Is there a specific club you could recommend?**

A   *I find Weightwatchers impressive and know a lot of people who have lost weight with them and kept it off. Sarah Ferguson, the Duchess of York, is a famous fan, although admittedly they pay her. Weightwatchers offers a well-balanced diet which uses a points system and no foods are forbidden. You can earn extra points for exercising, and you can hold them over until the following day, which is useful if you have a dinner date, for example. They have their own branded food which members are encouraged to use. This makes life easy, but I still prefer home cooking. Plenty of tips are given out during the meetings. Do check out who else operates near you. Most of the large organisations have online services too, but I think that personal contact works best.*

Q   Aren't all the people who go horribly competitive? Will I be the sad fat one at the back?

A   *Sometimes a little competition isn't a bad thing. As long as it doesn't get out of control – like spiking your rival's scales – it's good for motivation. Maybe you should take some support along with you. Would a friend or your partner come, for instance? Keep going and soon you'll be the slim one in the front.*

29

Snooze and lose

What has sleep got to do with weight loss? A lot more than you probably think. So get your pyjamas on. I'll tuck you in and explain.

One famous Hollywood actress allegedly owes her beauty and slender frame to very large amounts of sleep. Apparently it is not unusual for her to spend an entire 24 hours in bed, snoring away.

I'm sure that her personal chefs, trainers, makeup artists, hairdressers, acupuncturists, aromatherapists and all the other flunkies also play a part in maintaining her in peak physical condition, but the notion of sleep as a powerful aid to beauty and wellbeing makes perfect sense. As well as giving your body the time to recharge and repair itself, a good sleep makes you feel on top of the world. Just think how awful you feel without it: tired, lacking in concentration and energy, bad tempered and hungry. Research in the US has revealed that people who don't get enough sleep are more likely to go for high-sugar, high-fat foods and drink. The idea is that if you're not getting energy from rest, your body will encourage you to turn to quick-energy food.

Here's an idea for you...

Be careful with that coffee. Did you know a large full-fat latte packs in a hefty 260 calories? A cappuccino with skimmed milk has only 100 calories while black coffee is virtually calorie-free. Which one do you usually choose?

If you're not getting enough sleep on a prolonged basis, it could interfere with your body's ability to metabolise carbohydrates by up to 40%, according to another US study.

While we're asleep, our brains go through various stages, from stage one, which is light, drowsy sleep through to deep or slow-wave sleep and then on to Rapid Eye Movement (REM) sleep, in which our eyes move rapidly under our closed lids and our brain waves are active, although the body is paralysed. Experts generally agree that bodily repair happens in deep sleep and brain repair happens during REM sleep. You need both to be at your physical and mental best. Disruption of REM sleep has been found to lead to an increase in appetite.

HOW MUCH SLEEP DO YOU NEED?

This varies from person to person. Most of us sleep for between six and ten hours a night, with the average around eight hours. Whatever leaves you refreshed and full of energy to face the day is the right amount for you. As well as quantity, the quality of your sleep counts too and there are things you can do to maximise it. So if you've been feeling tired, sluggish and rather peckish all day, check your 'sleep hygiene' as the sleep scientists like to call it.

SIX SUGGESTIONS FOR BETTER SLEEP

■ Keep your bedroom for sleeping. Try not to
take work to bed, eat in bed or even watch
TV in bed. TV encourages snacking and also
doesn't create a restful atmosphere. Your
bedroom should be a comfortable temperature, dark and quiet.

■ Stimulants such as alcohol and caffeine are best avoided before bedtime as they
can cause twitching and tossing and turning. This might not wake you up, but it
will affect the quality of your sleep and leave you hungry for high calorie snacks
the next day.

■ Keep to a regular bedtime and waking up time whenever possible. If you're
sleeping badly, it might be worth forgetting the weekend lie-ins, since they will
interfere with your body's natural rhythm.

■ If your partner snores or next door's cats
like to serenade you at night, try earplugs.

■ When your mind races or you feel stressed
out and anxious, visualise yourself putting
your worries in a drawer and locking it, telling yourself you'll deal with it in the
morning. Or read a few chapters of a non-demanding book. Don't read anything
that will make you think too deeply or get agitated!

■ Make yourself a warm drink of milk (skimmed, of course). Although there's no
real proof this helps you feel sleepy, there's something very comforting about it.

**Omitting carbohydrates from
your diet can lead to sleep
problems. What are the other
pros and cons of high-protein,
low-carbohydrate diets? See
IDEA 40 *Trust me, I'm a doctor.***

Try another idea...

*'Early to bed and early to rise
makes a man healthy,
wealthy and wise.'*
BENJAMIN FRANKLIN

Defining idea...

123

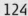

How did it go?

Q **I often get cramps in bed at night. Is it due to dieting? Am I lacking some nutrient?**

A *This is unlikely; actually cramps are usually thought to be a result of waste products collecting in the muscles because of poor circulation. Regular exercise can combat this, as well as burning up extra calories and so helping weight loss. You could also try this stretch: stand about a metre away from the wall and lean towards it, keeping your heels on the floor. Hold for 10–15 seconds and repeat.*

Q **What should I eat when I need an energy boost that won't wreck my diet?**

A *You could just try a brisk walk to revive yourself. Sometimes a change of scene is all that's needed. Or eat something that will provide a long-lasting boost, such as fruit, a wholemeal fruit scone, some low-fat cheese or a slice of chicken on a cracker or crispbread, or a bowl of low or no sugar cereal with skimmed milk. And remember, if you are getting sufficient and regular sleep and plenty of exercise, you may not need so many energy boosts anyway.*

30

What does it say on the label?

It has a little healthy eating logo on it, so it must be good for you, right? Reduced fat means I can eat a bigger portion too, doesn't it? No and no! Learn to read labels and help yourself lose weight.

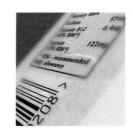

I'm something of a label freak and it's not just because I like a little bit of Gucci and Prada. If you read food labels, you can transform your body because you know much more about what you are eating.

It's not some nerdy hobby of mine. I had to start reading labels when my daughter was diagnosed as having a peanut allergy, as nuts can be hidden in all kinds of food and a reaction can be potentially fatal. Once you start reading labels, you discover interesting things – juice drinks with vegetable oils in them, for instance, or

Here's an idea for you... **Check the labels of various loaves of bread next time you're at the shops. Bread is a healthy food to eat, especially if it's wholemeal, but the fat content of a slice can vary quite dramatically between the brands, from around 60 calories a slice with 0.9 g of fat, to 115 calories a slice with 2.7 g of fat and even more!**

something you thought looked like a delicious fruity yoghurt that is just fruit-flavoured, not full of fruit. That 100 g (3.5 ounces) of your favourite cheddar cheese might turn out to add up to 410 calories and 34 g of fat.

As a starting point, you should know that food labels have to tell us things like the sell-by date and also state the country of origin. There has to be a list of ingredients too, with whatever the food or product contains most of named first and the rest listed in descending order. This is interesting when something looks full of meat, for example, and then you see that meat is actually the third thing listed rather than the first! Labels also give a nutritional breakdown, usually expressed per 100 g, but sometimes as a percentage of the RDA, which is the recommended daily amount suggested by the government and calculated to prevent nutritional deficiency in at least 95% of people. You can check the RDA against calories, fat, protein and so on. All of this is useful when you compare similar-seeming foods in the supermarket. It all becomes slightly more complicated when you start seeing extra little logos and words such 'lite' or 'reduced fat'. When you're trying to lose weight you're more conscious of these extra labels, but don't just take them at face value. Here's what they really mean:

■ **Lite/light** – Although manufacturers are encouraged to say what they mean by this, there are no real rules to say how much fat and how many calories should be in something that describes itself this way. The only way to work out whether it is as diet-friendly as it appears is to check the nutritional label yourself against a standard, i.e. non light, version. Check it against the per 100 g breakdown and you'll be able to judge for yourself what the difference is. Light in fat can still contain as many calories as a standard product because sugar has been added to compensate for example.

Think you might have a food allergy? Turn to IDEA 39, *I can't eat that because my allergy means it'll pile on pounds.*

Try another idea…

■ **Low fat/fat free** – By law you can't be misled on this one, but it's still not straightforward. The UK Food Standards Agency suggests to manufacturers that 'low fat' should only be claimed when the fat content is less than 3 g per 100 g. 'Fat-free' should be for foods that only have a trace of fat – under 0.15 mg per 100 g. Claims of '90% fat-free' used to be used quite freely and implied that it was perhaps a better bet than low fat. However, it basically meant that a food was still 10% fat – so it was actually not as good as low fat. Confused? Luckily, voluntary guidelines for labelling mean that this particular description is being used far less, but if you do see it, you have been warned!

■ **Reduced fat** – It sounds good, but the recommendation is that it can only appear on foods that have less than three quarters of the amount of fat of the standard product. Again, to really understand what you're getting, you'd have to

Defining
idea...

'It helps to know your labelling law here: a strawberry yoghurt must contain some strawberry. A strawberry-flavoured yoghurt has had a brief encounter with the fruit, while a strawberry flavour yoghurt has not even been within sight of a strawberry.'
FELICITY LAWRENCE, author of *Not on the Label*

check against the original product. Reduced fat taramasalata dip, for example, still contains 25 g fat per 100 g. So it's better than regular taramasalata, but not necessarily the best choice of dip (tomato-based salsa is an alternative).

Finally, beware 'healthy eating' style logos and labels. Quite often when fat is reduced in these types of products, fillers are used to bulk them up, and the sugar and salt contents may be high too. Maybe the calories are reduced because it's a tiny portion! As ever, do a comparative label check.

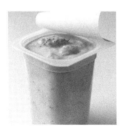
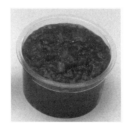
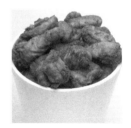

Q **If 3g per 100g is low fat, what is a lot of fat?**

A *As a rule of thumb, 20g of fat or more per 100g is a lot of fat.*

Q **What about organic foods? Aren't they healthier?**

A *Well, they certainly don't include as many additives which has to be healthier. Hydrogenated fats and artificial sweeteners are usually banned too, but they're not necessarily lower in fat or sugars (sugars can be 'natural'). Again, you really need to study the label closely to see what you're getting from a weight-loss perspective.*

Q **I've heard the term 'hidden sugars'. What are they and how can I spot them?**

A *These are simply sugars that are a little less obvious, i.e. you can't see them, or don't recognise the names they hide behind! They turn up in all sorts of things from burgers to baked beans. So as well as natural, raw and cane sugars, which are probably reasonably easy to spot, look for things ending in 'ose' – sucrose, lactose, dextrose and also malt extract, corn syrup, honey and molasses.*

How did it go?

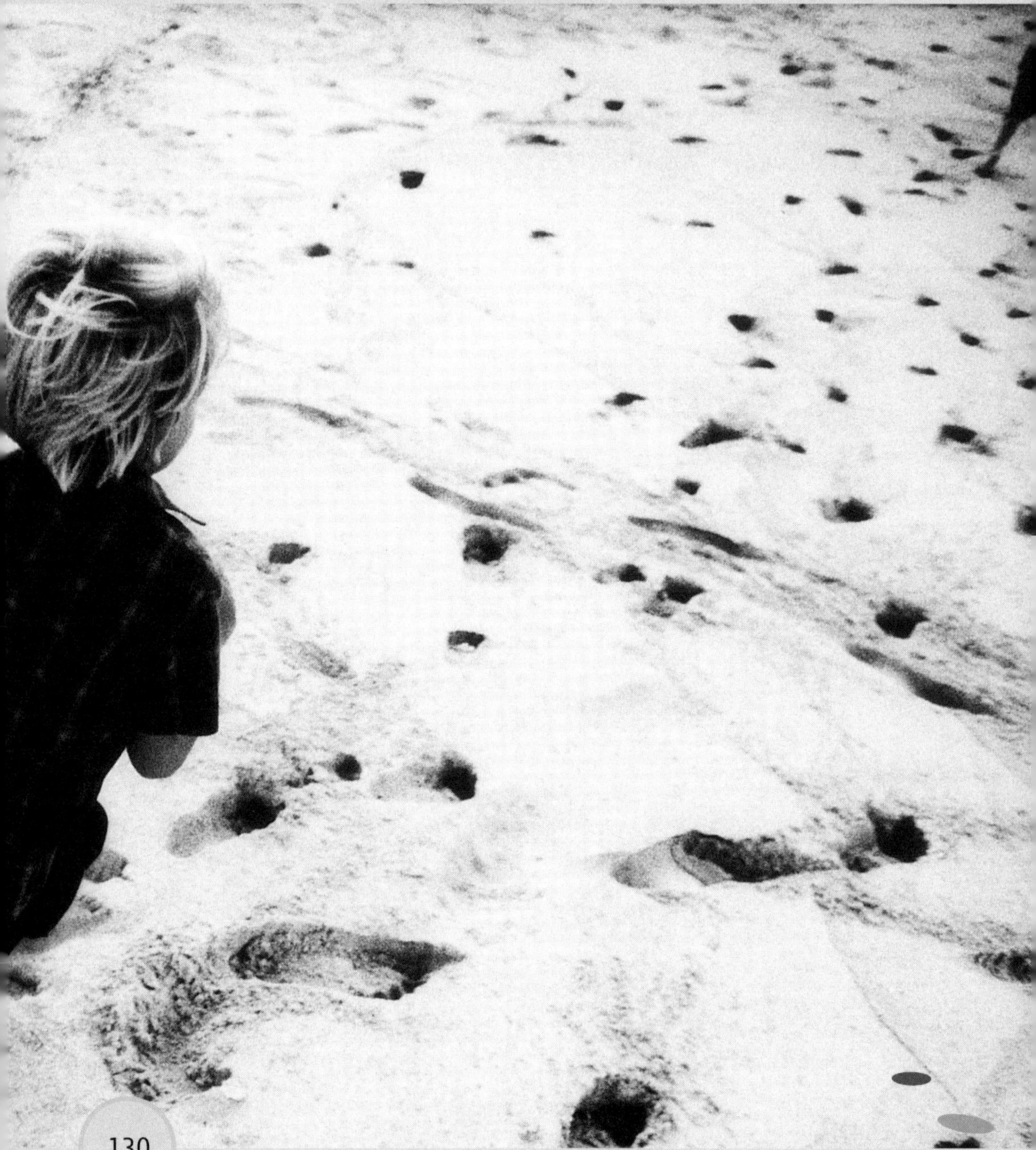

31

Easy ways to lose a pound a week without trying too hard

Simple food swaps, cutting back on high calorie treats and pushing yourself to be a little more active can help you achieve realistic, long-term weight loss. Mix and match these tips and you will look and feel slimmer with minimum effort.

There is always a less fattening choice of snack to be made, or a calorie-minimising way to cook. Take one of my favourite meals, the Caesar salad. It's a salad, so it must be good for you, right? Wrong!

Unfortunately, the Caesar salad has one of the most fattening dressings known to the hips, plus enough cheese and croutons to demand its own place setting at dinner. What can you do, apart from gaze at it longingly from across a crowded

Here's an idea for you...

Chew sugar-free gum or clean your teeth after a meal or a snack. As well as cleaning your teeth and giving you sweet breath, it sends you a psychological message that you have finished eating and that it is time to do something else. Make a clean break when your meal ends so that you really know that it is over.

room? You can make a lighter version, that's what. Just replace the fried croutons with baked ones, reduce the cheese drastically and go very light on the oil. There's always a solution, you see.

One of the best solutions to losing a little bit of weight every week is to make changes that are so simple, you'll barely notice them. It's safe and possible to lose half a kilo (a pound) a week if you shave 500 calories per day from your food intake (or expend it through activity). The maths behind this is that 3,500 calories equals half a kilo (a pound) of fat. So, divide 7 days into 3,500 and you get that magic 500 number. Do some more maths and you'll see that 500 g a week is 2 kg a month and 12 kg in six months. Get started with the following clever little ideas:

Say no to crisps

This is one of the most popular snacks, but a regular 40 g bag has around 200 calories and 10 g of fat. Even lighter versions come in at slightly over half of that amount. So if you stopped having a bag each day at work, you'd save at least 500 calories a week.

Avoid large portions

A large burger, fries and fizzy drink will easily stack up to 1000 calories, if not slightly more. If you can't cut them out, at least opt for the regular or small sizes which will cut the calories in half.

Watch what you drink

On a night out, three 175 ml glasses of white wine will cost you nearly 400 calories. Three spritzers will be half that. A half pint of strong lager clocks up around 160 calories, while a half of ordinary strength is about 80 calories. Steer clear of cocktails too – a pina colada is easily 225 calories, while a vodka and slimline tonic is just 60.

On your bike

Eco-friendly, fun and jolly good exercise, an hour's cycling should take care of nearly 500 calories.

Sandwich swap

If you have a little low fat salad cream in your lunchtime sandwich instead of lashings of butter, you could save up to 500 calories during your working week.

Rethink your Saturday night take-away

Choose chicken chow mein and boiled rice over sweet and sour chicken and fried rice, you'll save around 500 calories.

Walk more

If you walk to work, the shops or just for fun (but at a reasonably brisk pace) you'll burn up around 250 calories an hour.

Got a sweet tooth? Try IDEA 17 _Sweet temptation._

Try another idea...

'*Another good reducing exercise consists of placing both hands against the table edge and pushing back.*'
ROBERT QUILLEN

Defining idea...

Wash the car

Save money and burn energy by valeting your car. Wash it, polish it and vacuum it inside and you'll use up a few hundred calories,

Have a skinnier coffee

You could save yourself 170 calories if you opted for a regular white coffee, made with skimmed milk, rather than a cappuccino made with full fat milk.

Party snacks

Think such small little nibbles don't count? If you had two tablespoons of tzatziki dip that would add up to around 40 calories. Two tablespoons of taramasalata, however, is 130 calories. Thick meat pate on French bread can cost you about 250 calories, whereas a small helping of smoked salmon on rye bread is a mere 130 calories. A cocktail sausage is around 70 calories. Wrap it in pastry and serve it as a sausage roll and you're looking at 200 calories.

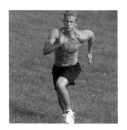 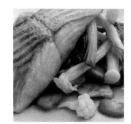 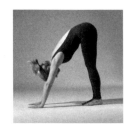

Q   My weakness is cheese. How can I lose weight and still indulge?

A   Keep your portion sizes matchbox small and enjoy a delicious ripe piece of fruit with it. Some cheeses are also more heavyweight than others. Cheddar, for example, is around 124 calories per 30 g with around 10 g of fat. The same weight of camembert is about 90 calories with 7 g of fat, while feta is 75 calories and 6 g of fat. Check labels to make comparisons and the best choices. You could also try grating cheese to have on toast or a cracker rather than slicing it, so you still get the taste, only fewer calories.

Q   I'm too busy to walk or cycle, so I can't really burn up extra energy that way, can I?

A   Ultimately you're going to have to find a way to schedule some exercise into your life. You could start by breaking it down into smaller chunks. For example, if you took half an hour's walking a day as your target, you could break it down into three ten minute sessions, say a walk before breakfast, one at lunchtime and one in the evening. I don't think that's impossible for anyone.

Q   Does it help you lose weight if you don't eat after 6 p.m.?

A   There isn't a proven link between eating in the evening and gaining weight. You might eat more over dinner, especially if you eat out, but your metabolism isn't slowing down as dusk falls. It does when you're asleep though!

How did it go?

135

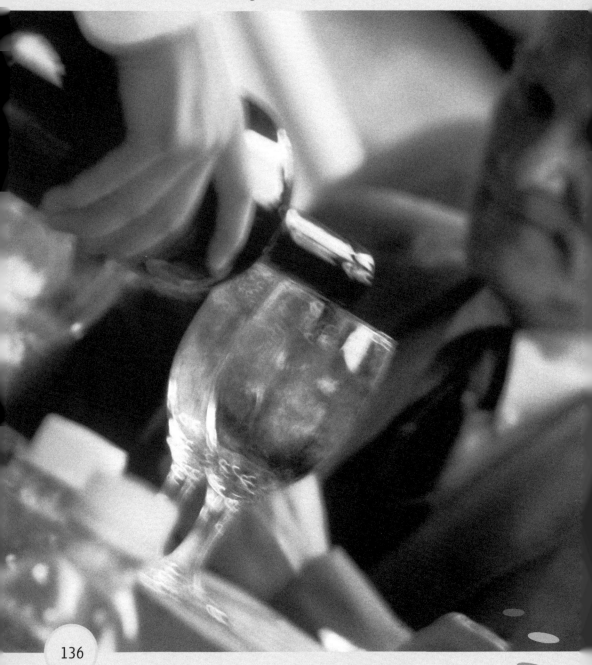

32

High spirits

Sociable, mood-enhancing, delicious ... but alcohol can also be ruinous to your diet. When should you call time on your drinking?

Some diets expressly ban alcohol. Others allow you a few measures a week. Personally I follow the 'everything in moderation' school. The point is that if you deprive yourself of too much, you won't keep up with your programme.

The trouble with alcohol is that one glass so easily leads to another. Or four. And that's where the problems can lie.

The UK recommended guidelines for alcohol consumption are 21 units for men and 14 for women. These are quite conservative recommendations, so a few extra units every now and then won't pose any serious health risk. You do need to be unit-aware. A unit is always disappointingly small, I think – a half pint of beer, a small (125 ml) glass of wine and a single measure (25 ml) of spirits. Often, it's hard to keep track of how many units you've had, especially if you are drinking at home or

Here's an idea for you...

If you're eating out, save the alcohol for during the meal rather than tucking in to the aperitifs too. As well as cutting back a few calories, this will leave you with a clear head when you come to order. Alcohol can have a strange way of making deep fried camembert or kalamari look like the perfect choice for dieters!

ordering say a 'large' glass of wine in a restaurant. Some restaurants appear to be serving up half a bottle of wine in a glass these days, which might seem good value for money but can stack up to four units and a few hundred calories. Interestingly, doctors reckon that people underestimate their alcohol consumption by 50%, which is why it's a good idea to record your intake over a period of a few weeks to assess if you need to make some changes. The health dangers of excess alcohol include liver damage, mood swings and malnutrition. Of course, regularly drinking to excess requires professional help. It's estimated that a regular daily intake of eight units by men and six by women can lead to long-term damage, with 20% of heavy drinkers going on to develop cirrhosis of the liver. Spreading your alcohol consumption over a week, rather than binge drinking is thought to be healthier for the liver, not to mention your head. Try to keep a few days alcohol-free too.

ALCOHOL AND DIET

Alcohol is full of calories, which gives the body an instant energy hit, but not much else, as alcohol has few nutrients to boast about. If you calculate that in order to lose a pound a week, you need to cut 500 calories a day – 3500 calories make half a kilo (a pound), which, divided by the seven days of the week, equals 500. A strong lager can clock up 350 calories, so it's not hard to understand why cutting down on alcohol makes sense. Then there's the fact that alcohol seems to make you snack. How quickly handfuls of peanuts and crisps slip down when you're enjoying a few cocktails! How much easier is it to have a burger or huge ham, cheese and mayonnaise sandwich after a few drinks than start cooking yourself something healthy?! And while there are a few people who can't face food the morning after the night before, the majority of us just can't help feeding a hangover. There's no doubt that alcohol weakens the resolve, so resolve to keep it under control.

Try another idea...

It's hard to resist free-flowing drinks and canapés when you're in the party mood. But how do you deal with falling off the diet bandwagon? See IDEA 25 *The morning after the night before.*

There are less fattening choices of drinks of course. If you have a white wine spritzer instead of a large (175 ml) glass of wine, i.e. use half the amount of wine and top up with soda or carbonated water you will save half the calories. Strong lagers are usually twice as high in calories as ordinary strength lagers. Slimline or diet mixers will also help to reduce the calorific impact of tipples such as vodka and tonic. So you can save calories and still have a good time!

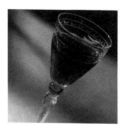

Defining idea...

'Only Irish coffee provides in a single glass all four essential food groups: alcohol, caffeine, sugar and fat.'
ALEX LEVINE

How did it go?

Q   I'm always reading that wine is really good for you. Is this true?

A   *Research has suggested that wine, and red wine in particular, can help protect against heart disease and stroke. More recently, it was discovered that an antioxidant in red wine, reservatrol, also protects against lung diseases. Most of the evidence is slightly skewed to favour middle-aged and elderly men, more than younger men and women though. The best advice is to stick within the recommended safe units and enjoy, rather than thinking you're doing yourself any great health favours!*

Q   I find it difficult to stop at just one glass of wine. Just as with biscuits, I open a packet and eat the lot. I can easily sink a bottle by myself.

A   *Me too. Addictive personality or just plain greedy, who knows? There is of course a health issue here. If you're doing that often, you could develop quite a serious alcohol problem. But on a lighter note, one way to deal with this is to buy expensive wine and create a bit of a ritual around it. Decant it or put it in an ice bucket. Promise yourself you will really enjoy two glasses only. Wait until an appointed hour and the drink it slowly and savour it. Have some food with it too. If you're out, designate yourself the driver, so you can't drink more than a glass or two.*

33

Stop the middle-age spread!

As you get older, gaining weight is easier and losing weight is harder. Here are a couple of common reasons why, and what you can do about them.

Previous generations accepted that a few bulges in all the wrong places was just what happened as you aged. But in our far more lookist, sizeist, ageist society, that just won't do.

There's no doubt that after the age of about thirty it gets much harder to shake off excess weight. This is particularly annoying if you don't think you're overeating. There could be some very good reasons why this is happening, as well as some good excuses. The key is to identify the potential physiological changes that apply to you personally and act on them.

Here's an idea for you... **Set the table, draw the curtains, light some candles and enjoy a leisurely supper. Your environment can have a huge impact on how much you eat. The noisy, colourful atmosphere in fast food restaurants and cafes stimulates the appetite. Try to relax over your food in a more subdued atmosphere.**

COULD YOU HAVE A THYROID PROBLEM?

An underactive thyroid (hypothyroidism) is a common condition, especially in women, with two in every hundred experiencing problems. Its classic symptom is weight gain.

The thyroid gland controls the body's metabolic processes, how quickly calories are burned up and how energy is used. When you have an underactive thyroid, your metabolism will be sluggish, you'll probably feel tired and low and you may have poor concentration. Other symptoms include high blood pressure and muscle and joint pain. A blood test will reveal the condition, which is treated with thyroxine (one of the thyroid hormones). If you suspect you have a thyroid problem, see your doctor.

IS STRESS MAKING YOU FAT?

Some people barely eat anything when they're under pressure, so the weight falls off them. For most of us, though, the opposite is true. This is not simply to do with the comfort eating and extra snacking that we indulge in when we're wound up. It seems there is hormonal connection to stress which causes a certain kind of weight gain.

Our bodies react with the 'fight or flight' response when we're under pressure. In Stone Age this was helpful when, say, we were being attacked by a wild animal, but today we can just as easily feel like this when we're late for an important meeting and stuck in a traffic jam. The body responds to a stressful scenario by saying, 'OK we need extra fuel here to cope', and releases the hormone cortisol, which helps us to use glucose stores for fuel. The cortisol stays in the bloodstream after the stress levels have calmed down, continuing to stimulate the appetite to replenish the glucose stores. So, stress makes your body want food, even though it hasn't actually burned off any extra calories. The result? Weight gain. Some experts also say that cortisol-related weight is stored around the abdomen, rather than thighs and buttocks, which is not a good place to store fat because of its association with heart disease.

A glass of wine after work or biscuits with a cup of tea will mount up to extra calories! Keeping track of what you're eating (and where you're sabotaging your dieting efforts) is easy with a food diary as explained in IDEA 6 *Get the write habit.*

Try another idea...

If it sounds as if it could be happening to you, try two things. First, make sure that you have a good supply of healthy snacks in anticipation of stressful moments. If you've got chocolate, crisps and pies around, that's what you'll eat. If you have crudités, wholemeal rolls with a healthy filling, fruit and so on, they will satisfy your stressed-out urges just as well. In the longer term you need to find ways of dealing with that stress through exercise, massage, therapy or maybe even a serious life change.

We can always make plenty of excuses for why we have put weight on and why we can't shift it. Think about the real reasons you are in this situation. Is your life very sedentary? Do you eat enormous portions? Do you snack on confectionery without even noticing? If you're making excuses to yourself all the time, you'll never reach your goals.

'Several excuses are always less convincing than one.'
ALDOUS HUXLEY

Defining idea...

*How did
it go?*

Q **My lifestyle is sedentary and I know it's not helping my efforts to slim down. How can I start getting more active?**

A *Why not try the 'three minutes an hour' rule? Once an hour, get up and walk, skip, dance, run up and down the stairs or whatever else you can think of for at least three minutes. Over the course of a day, it should add up to a minimum of thirty minutes, which is getting towards the amount you need to do to start seeing and feeling some of the benefits of exercise.*

Q **I'm always eating on the run, so end up grabbing high calorie snacks. How do I stop?**

A *Try to make healthier choices. Could you prepare your food at home and take it with you? Make it a rule to always sit at a table, chew slowly and taste what you're eating. That way, you can get back in touch with your body and its relationship with food.*

Q **I work in a high pressure job which I enjoy, but I realise it could be affecting my weight. Are there any instant de-stressing ideas?**

A *If you can get outside for just five minutes and be in some green space, or even just look at a window box, you'll reduce stress levels, lower your blood pressure and feel clear and focused, according to US research.*

34

Suck it out: the surgical route to fat loss

An alternative to dieting or the icing on the cake when you've lost weight and need a boost? It's not without risks, so here's what you need to know about cosmetic surgery.

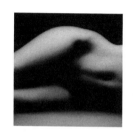

If you don't like your long toes, you can get them shortened. You can swap an 'outie' belly button for an 'innie'. You can even buy J Lo's bottom for yourself.

Cosmetic surgery has come a long way. It is now possible to sculpt away that excess fat. The downside is that it's expensive, it isn't always successful and it might not make you any happier. Surgery is not a good alternative to eating less and being active, which is the safe and sensible approach to weight control. Personally, I do feel that surgery is a last resort, but if you have lost lots of weight and the fat loss has left you with loose rolls of skin, a tummy tuck might give you a confidence boost. The most important thing is to do lots of research, ask questions and find the best possible surgeon.

Try an instant image change with a haircut. Layers can make your face look slimmer as can highlights. For men, a short, sharp haircut can make you look more George Clooney than Billy Bunter. Great hair works wonders.

Any surgery carries risks, such as infections, bleeding and reactions to anaesthetic. It's also important to see several surgeons before committing yourself to a procedure and ask them plenty of questions, including the following:

■ How often have you performed the procedure?

■ What kind of anaesthetic is used and who will administer it?

■ How long will the procedure take and how long will the results last?

■ Where will the incisions be and what level of scarring might I be left with?

■ What's the recovery time?

■ Can I see 'before and after' pictures and testimonials from other patients?

WHAT SURGERY IS ON OFFER?

One option for fat removal is liposuction, where a narrow metal tube is inserted into the fatty area via an incision in your skin. The surgeon moves the tube back and forth and sucks out the fat with a vacuum pump, leaving the nerves and blood vessels intact. There are variations in techniques, but that's the general idea. There is a maximum amount of fat that can be removed from an area, so you might not be able to sculpt off as much as you like. It also doesn't affect cellulite (the lumpy, dimply bane of many women's lives) and can leave skin loose. Following the procedure, your skin usually retracts and is bruised and uncomfortable. Healing can take a long time, with lumpiness and swelling taking up to six months to disappear. It's definitely not for the faint-hearted. Neither is a tummy tuck (abdominoplasty). With this procedure, excess skin and fat can be removed and muscles tightened. There are mini, standard and extended versions. All leave a scar, from a low one at the level of the pubic hair to one that extends around to the back. Are you feeling faint at this point? Me too, but let me tell you about a couple of new developments. The latest high-tech techniques include LipoSelection by Vaser, which uses advanced ultrasound technology to separate out the fatty tissue from the rest before it is removed. This is claimed to be more precise, gentler and less painful, with a quicker recovery time. There is also the lower body lift, which pulls up all your slack skin around the hips, thighs and stomach. It is claimed to smooth out cellulite, flattening lumpy 'orange-peel' skin. You can also get arm and breast lifts, and just in case your hands don't match your newly slim and lifted body, there is now plenty that can be done, from getting rid of bulging veins to plumping up saggy hand skin with your very own recycled bottom fat! Excuse me, I must go and lie down as I'm feeling rather queasy.

> Enough of fat in our bodies (and having it sucked out). What you really need to know about is fat in food. Learn more in IDEA 9, *Fats: the good, the bad and the downright ugly.*

Try another idea...

> '*I was going to have cosmetic surgery until I noticed that the doctor's office was full of portraits by Picasso.*'
> RITA RUDNER

Defining idea...

How did it go?

Q   How much do these sorts of operations cost?

A   *Prices depend on individual surgeons and hospitals, and the specific techniques used. However, the cost of a tummy tuck and liposuction would probably pay for gym membership, a personal trainer, a nutritionist and goodness knows what else for at least a year.*

Q   How do I find a surgeon?

A   *As well as seeking out personal recommendations, check that they are members of a professional body such as The British Association of Aesthetic Plastic Surgeons (BAAPS). New BAAPS members, for example, have to be recommended by two others who are aware of their ability, skills and knowledge.*

Q   Is there such a thing as a toe job?

A   *Yes. It involves making little incisions, cutting a bit of bone out, then reattaching the tendon. Result? Prettier toes.*

35

Shape up from home

While cash undoubtedly helps, you don't have to join an expensive gym to lose weight and get fit. If you're motivated, there's plenty you can do from home.

There are lots of little things you can do around the house to be more active. Everything counts, even hiding the TV remote control so you have to get up to change channels and the volume.

To really burn calories and see a difference in your body, the level of activity has to be revved up a few notches. For many people, exercising from home is the ideal solution, as it fits in with almost any lifestyle and can work for every budget. Here are some ideas to get you started:

FITNESS VIDEOS

These are very cost effective, provided you use them regularly and don't simply file them beside your complete collection of Bond movies. Go for a variety so that you don't get bored too quickly, and choose whatever you think looks like fun, whether

Here's an idea for you... **If you've been running for a while and enjoy it, why not join a running club to keep your motivation high? Or you could sign up for a charity fun run, such as the Race for Life series. Or dare you think about training for a marathon? Check out www.coolrunning.com.**

it's dance-inspired or a celebrity fat-burner. Make sure that at least one of them has a body sculpting or resistance training section so that you get all-round benefits. For the resistance training you'll need to use stretchy bands or dumbbells, which are available at sports shops and some department stores. In an emergency you can use a can of beans or bag of sugar in each hand instead!

Do the resistance training section of a fitness video two or three times a week and the faster, more aerobic section three to five times a week. After just a few weeks you should notice that it's getting easier and that you're starting to firm up. If not, have you just been sitting on the sofa watching it? As your new eating habits and the exercise work together, your body fat will gradually decrease.

A HOME CIRCUIT

With just a few pieces of equipment, you can set up your own version of a fitness circuit. All you need are a skipping rope, a mat or a couple of thick towels to protect your joints from cold, hard surfaces, some stairs and a resistance band such as a Dyna-Band, which comes with an illustrated sheet of exercises, .

Start with a warm up by walking up and down the stairs or around the block. Next, skip or stair-step for one minute, followed by twenty repetitions of a toning exercise from the resistance band sheet such as an upper body exercise. Then, do your minute's aerobic exercise again, followed by another toning session. This time, do a lower body move or some stomach exercises. Continue the circuit for about fifteen minutes and aim to do it twice a week. To progress, all you need to do are more repetitions or different toning exercises and longer aerobics sections. Add a purely cardiovascular activity to the two sessions of circuit training and you'll be slimmer and more toned in just a few weeks.

For another exercise idea that's easy to fit in to any lifestyle, look at IDEA 19, *Walk yourself thinner.*

Try another idea...

RUNNING

This is a fantastic way to burn fat, tone your legs and boost your fitness. Running requires a good pair of running shoes and comfy clothing; do go to a specialist sports shop to get them. An easy way to start is to walk for a few minutes, then run for a few minutes, then walk again and so on. As you progress, you'll be running more and walking less! You could also invest in a heart monitor which transmits your heart rate to a wrist display, to check you're working at the right level. To burn fat you need to work at about 70% of your maximum heart rate – make that a goal for later if you're just starting out, rather than trying to do it straight away. To work out your maximum heart rate, subtract your age from 220 and multiply that figure by 0.7. Another way to check if you're running too hard is if you're unable to speak! It's better to run, jog or even walk more slowly for longer, than it is to go hell for leather and collapse in a heap after ten minutes.

'The best thing about running is that it can give you whatever you need – whether that's a better body, quiet time to think, or something more radical like the confidence to make life-changing decisions or tackle an "I didn't think I had it in me" challenge.'
SUSIE WHALLEY and LISA JACKSON, *Running Made Easy*

Defining idea...

How did
it go?

Q   **I've got a couple of fitness videos, but how can I find the time to do them?**

A   Schedule time for exercise, just as you note down an appointment in your diary. It might sound pedantic, but it should ensure you take your efforts seriously! Remember you don't have to do the whole video in one go. You could do one section in the morning and one in the evening, or one today and one tomorrow. The key is to keep doing something and build on your success.

Q   **I think I've reached a fitness plateau. How do I know if what I'm doing is worth it?**

A   Why not try a personal training session? A trainer can gear workouts to your needs and goals and help with motivation. Just a few sessions can put you on the right track again.

Q   **I was thinking of buying a mini trampoline to work out on at home. What do you think?**

A   These are great for injury rehabilitation because they reduce the stress on the joints. However, if you're uninjured, it is hard to work vigorously enough to improve your cardiovascular fitness on a trampoline. Impact activities like jogging, aerobics and so on are good for improving bone density, which is something you wouldn't get bouncing on your trampoline. If you think it will be fun and it will get you to do something, then go ahead. If you're already exercising regularly, though, save the money for a new pair of trainers or personal training session instead.

36

Dieting danger

Disordered eating is frightening, confusing and poses severe health risks. While the causes are complex and not fully understood, everyone should be aware of the danger signs of eating habits that are getting out of control.

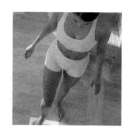

Contrary to popular belief, eating disorders are not a modern illness — they have been going on for centuries. What is true, is that they now seem to be on the increase.

Much disordered eating is kept secret until it becomes patently obvious that there's a problem, so it is hard to put any real figures on how many sufferers there really are. More and more people are coming forward for help and treatment for themselves or their friends and family members.

Eating disorders are difficult to understand, whether you're a sufferer or watching someone else suffer, but I think it is especially hard on the latter group. Why does someone who has starved themselves still insist they're fat? What is going on in the mind of someone who looks perfectly gorgeous yet steals away to the bathroom a few times a week to vomit? How can they be ashamed of what they've eaten and afraid to gain weight when they are obviously thin?

Here's an idea for you... **Get yourself along to a self help group. Talking to others who have experienced the same issues and problems and can offer support and understanding without blaming you or making you feel guilty, can be a real help.**

Some experts think there is a link between dieting and developing eating disorders, especially bulimia. The theory goes that dieting makes you hungry, which makes you binge, which then makes you feel guilty. In susceptible people, a purge (vomiting or using laxatives), helps to deal with the guilt and 'remove' the calories.

There are millions of us who diet without developing these kinds of illnesses. What has been discovered is that people who have eating disorders also share certain personality traits – they are perfectionists, who are eager to please, yet who have low self-esteem. When these factors are combined with family troubles (divorce, bereavement) or indeed certain family attitudes to weight and food, the spiral into illness can be quick. Ultimately, eating disorders are usually about control.

Treatment is available, but success is dependent on the individual accepting help. Even then, there are a proportion of people who will continue to obsess about weight and food for the rest of their lives. Anorexics will usually be referred to a specialist psychiatrist who is experienced in eating disorders, which may be enough to get attitudes to food and eating back to somewhere approaching healthy. However, some anorexics will be hospitalised because of the lack of fluids and nutrients in their bodies, which is even more distressing, not only for the carers, but for the sufferer themselves as they feel themselves losing what little control they have in their lives. For bulimics, anti-depressants have been found to help reduce bingeing, but psychological treatment is essential too.

Check whether your own eating habits and attitudes, or those of a friend or family member, could indicate signs of disordered eating. If you're concerned, see your doctor, contact a self-help group or check The Eating Disorders Association at www.edauk.com.

Focus on developing a healthy body image. Turn to IDEA 11, With friends like you, who needs enemies?

Try another idea...

The following is not an exhaustive list, but some common indications that issues exist or are beginning to develop include:

- Not eating in front of others, claiming to have just eaten or having prepared a meal for others.

- Being secretive around food

- A strong fear of gaining weight, although you have an acceptable weight or are even underweight.

- Distorted body image – believing you're fat when you're at an acceptable weight or underweight

- Recurrent bingeing – eating too much in a short space of time, i.e. within a few hours.

'It's important to remember that eating disorders are very complex conditions and are not about dieting going too far. The vast majority of people who diet don't have eating disorders.'
LYNDEL COSTAIN, *Diet Trials: How to Succeed at Dieting*

Defining idea...

■ Shame and guilt after eating leading to using laxatives, or making yourself vomit

■ Obsession with exercise – working out several times a day for a couple of hours at a time

■ Judging yourself solely on looks

■ Ritualistic eating habits such as cutting food into tiny pieces

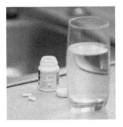 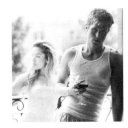 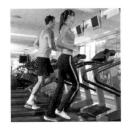

Q **I think about food all the time, especially about what I've just eaten and what I'll eat next. I don't have a problem, do I?**

How did it go?

A *Maybe not, but it doesn't sound as though your relationship with food is all that healthy either. Sorry to sound nannyish, but you could probably use some professional support, via a nutritionist or friendly doctor.*

Q: **I have a friend who has dieted as long as I've known her. I'm sure she's anorexic but she gets really angry if I try to talk to her about it. What can I do?**

A *Of course you want to help, but often this will be perceived as criticism or pressure which will only make things worse. All you can do is be there, listen, love and support. Once your friend has recognised she has a problem, you can lend practical support in finding help, going along to medical appointments and so on.*

Q **I binge, but don't vomit or use laxatives. So I'm ok, aren't I?**

A *Many binge eaters eat to escape their emotions, but then feel that food makes them out of control. If you binge but don't purge, you may well also be very overweight. Medical help is essential to get you out of this behaviour. Pluck up the courage to ask for it. You won't regret it.*

157

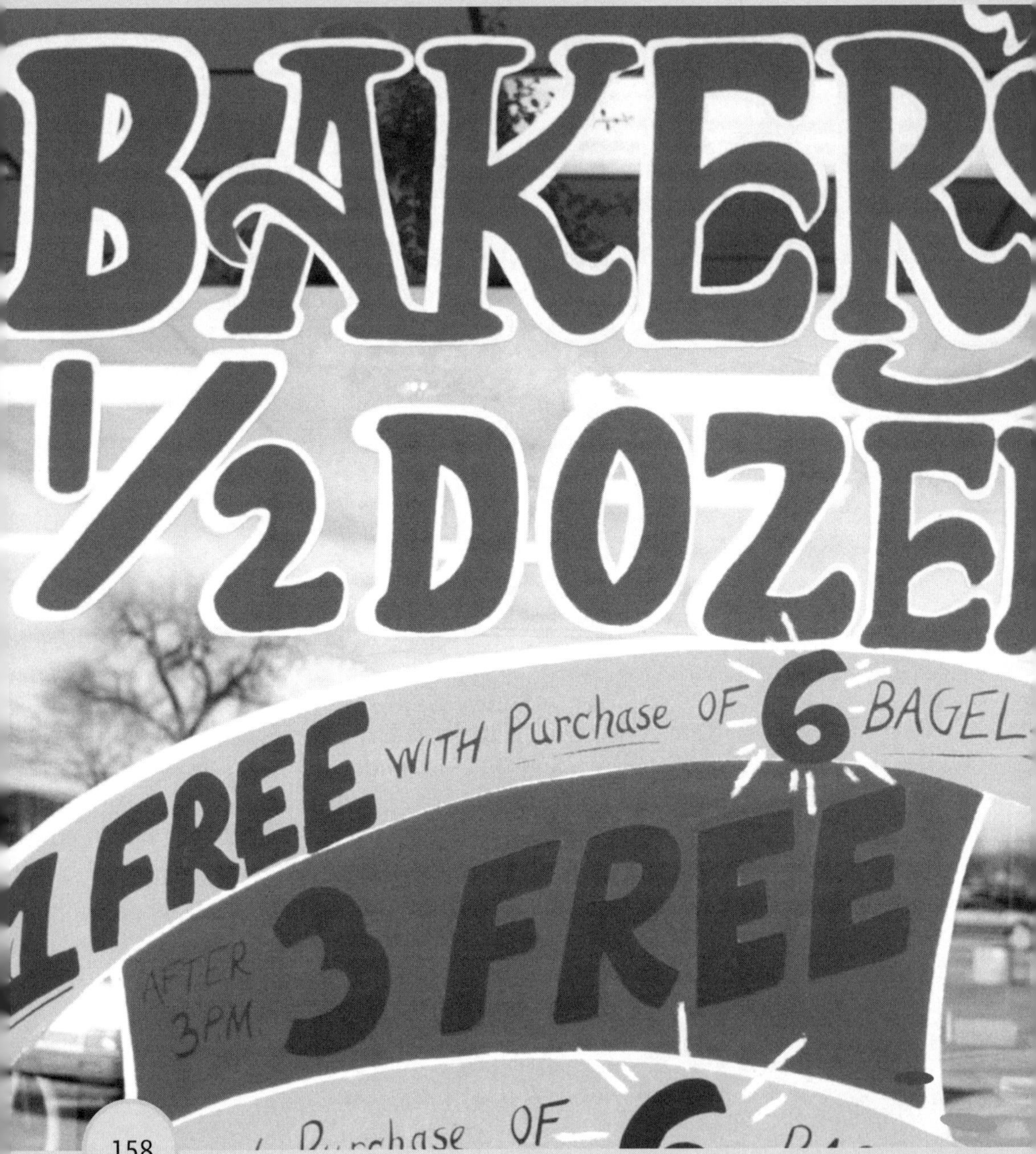
BAKER
½ DOZE
1 FREE WITH Purchase OF 6 BAGEL
AFTER 3PM.
3 FREE
Purchase OF

37

How to be smart (slim) shopper

You can save yourself pounds (£s and lbs!) by shopping wisely. Here are a few tricks to help you make the leanest deals and find the best buys for your thighs.

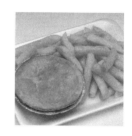

Good intentions are a commendable thing, but soon lose their rose-tinted glow if that's all they remain. Translate them into action, and keep going.

Losing weight means getting on and doing it, not just thinking about it. It means being prepared, which is where being a savvy shopper comes in. What's the point of deciding you'll prepare a delicious low-fat meal if all you have in the house is some ready-made pastry, a string of sausages and some out-of-date double cream? How can you protect yourself from a snack attack when all your larder contains is a family-sized bag of crisps? Shopping for food might well be a chore, but haphazard shopping will cost you dear in the weight-loss stakes. Here are some things to think about:

Here's an idea for you... **Chop bananas into bite-sized chunks and freeze them. They then become healthy, delicious, almost ice-creamy treats to snack on. You can freeze grapes too or make your own ice lollies by freezing fruit juice.**

Do not go shopping when you're hungry. Your eyes will be seduced by all the high-fat, calorie-rich possibilities on offer, while your body says "feed me, I'm hungry, feed me now". This will get you thinking about an impromptu picnic in the supermarket car park, so have a meal or snack before you go. Take a list too. That way, you'll buy everything you really need and minimise the threat of impulse buys . Let's be honest, no one buys extra cabbage on impulse – you know the sort of temptations I'm really referring to.

If you can, plan some easy, healthy meals you can cook yourself and shop for the fresh ingredients. Get away from an over-reliance on convenience foods and slash fat and calories from your diet. Even if they have a healthy eating or reduced fat logo, check the labels to see what you're really getting. Low fat only counts if it is 3 g or less per 100 g. Avoid special offers, super-sizes and multi-buys unless they're healthy and low fat. Short of wearing a mask over your eyes and nose, it's difficult not to notice the lovely aromas and free samples all around you so you just have to accept that supermarkets are run by clever people who want to sell you lots of things. Even the way they lay out their stores is a cunning ploy to ensure you see everything they offer. As well as the tips above, you have to be strong and say "No thanks, not today". A trip around the aisles should end up looking something like this:

IN THE TROLLEY

Fill it up with:

- Wholegrains – they're not less calorific than white, refined produce, but they have more fibre and will keep you feeling full for longer

- Lots of colourful fruit and vegetables

- Low-fat dairy produce

- Lean cuts of meat, chicken and turkey (the white meat is lower in fat than dark)

- Fish, including a portion or two of oily fish, such as salmon, tuna, mackerel and herring

- Dried fruit to snack on – it's calorific, but OK if you keep servings small; low-fat/reduced-calorie cereal

- Low-fat and cereal snack bars – but still check the label for the better buys

Done the shopping and missed your opportunity to do an exercise class? You need help with your support network. See **IDEA 51, Support act.**

Try another idea...

'I can spend hours in a grocery store. I get so excited when I see food, I go crazy.'
CAMERON DIAZ

Defining idea...

161

THINGS TO LEAVE ON THE SHELF

- Cereals with added sugar (pick out the sugar free ones and choose oats if you like porridge or making your own muesli)

- Biscuits and cakes, crisps

- Sausages, meat pies and pasties

- Anything with pastry

- Battered and bread-crumbed meat and seafood (all that extra fat and calories)

- Sugary jams and spreads (choose sugar-free versions)

- Full fat ice-cream – why not try frozen yoghurt instead?

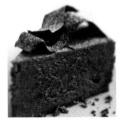 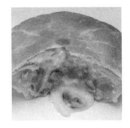 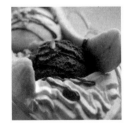

Q   **I need another snack idea. Do you have any?**

A   *Try making your own popcorn. Buy your corn kernels and add 50 g to a saucepan in which you've heated one tablespoon of oil. Put the lid on, and they'll pop in a few minutes. You can experiment with flavours. If you have a sweet tooth, try adding some cinnamon or grated orange rind. For a savoury snack, add curry powder, black pepper or garlic powder. It's tasty, low fat, high fibre and has a few B vitamins.*

Q   **Any other tips for distraction? I'm not sure I can make it past the cake counter in one piece.**

A   *Perhaps you could start viewing your shopping trip as part of your daily exercise plan. Buy a pedometer, which measures how many steps you're taking and how many calories you're burning. 10,000 steps a day, which is not as hard to achieve as it sounds, will go a long way to keeping you fit and healthy.*

Q   **I shall get bored with grilled chicken breasts for the rest of my life, won't I?**

A   *I think you're being over-dramatic. There are lots of easy, healthy, low fat cook books out there to inspire you. Besides, you could get creative with store cupboard condiments alongside your grills. Have you ever heard of salsa, mustard, balsamic vinegar, horseradish and chutney? Have some fun and surprise yourself!*

How did it go?

163

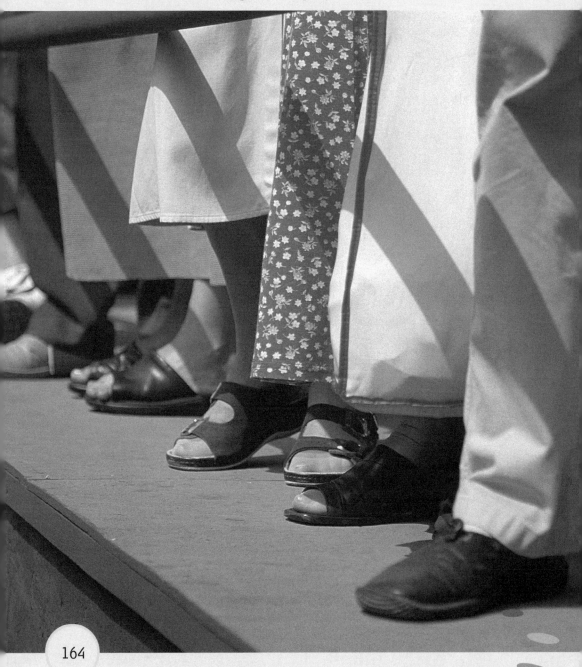

38

Alternatives to kaftans

Being groomed and stylish is confidence-boosting whether you're just starting out on your weight loss plan or already beginning to change shape.

As well as looking good, it will make you feel good about yourself. A few sartorial tricks will go a long way to making you appear thinner than you are.

Stylish, streamlined dressing isn't a question of size or money, despite the famous remark of Wallis Simpson, the Duchess of Windsor, that 'one can never be too thin or too rich'. The extraordinary amount of choice on the high street now means that whatever your budget or measurements, you'll be able to find clothes that suit you. It wasn't ever thus. Not so long ago, unless you were a 'size tiny', all that was on offer was a tent, a kaftan or baggy tracksuit. Manufacturers and retailers have woken up at last to the fact that people come in all shapes and sizes and want to look good. Of course, it's not just what you wear, it's the way that you wear it too. Here are some super-useful tips for dressing well and dressing to look slimmer:

Here's an idea for you... **Go through your wardrobe and throw away anything that is baggy and shapeless or too tight. Try on doubtful items and take a long hard look at yourself in the mirror. Does it flatter you? Any doubts, chuck it out.**

FOR WOMEN

- To disguise a big belly, don't wear your tops tucked in. Try a chunky low slung belt worn over a loose top.

- An A-line skirt is great for hiding big thighs and bottoms.

- Combat trousers and narrow tight-fitting trousers will maximise every curve. Try a boot leg cut or flares to take the emphasis away from a large top half.

- Keep detail simple. Lots of pockets, buttons, bows, prints and zips look over-fussy and can make you appear wider.

- If you have a large bust and arms, say no to thin spaghetti straps and ruffle necks. Keep it simple with tailored shirts and jackets and v necks.

- A long jacket hides a fuller figure. Boxy jackets just make you look square-shaped.

- Beware anything that is too small – and this includes your underwear – as you will just bulge out.

- Go for fabrics that drape, such as cotton, lightweight knits and jerseys as opposed to fabrics that cling, such as satin and Lycra.

- Skirts that end just below the knee tend to make your legs look longer.

For more on body shapes, go to IDEA 47, *Spot reduction: the facts and the fiction.*

Try another idea...

- Beware of shoes with ankle straps, which have the effect of cutting off your legs and shortening them. Heels are great for extra height and leg lengthening, as are boots. If you have big calves, go for boots in a stretchy material. They go with practically anything.

- Wearing one colour, or complementary tones of a colour streamlines your body. As a general rule, darker colours are more slimming.

- Leggings and other Lycra trousers and shorts should be kept for the gym.

- Wide-legged trousers flatter pear-shapes. Trousers that do up on the side will also minimise a belly and bottom.

FOR MEN

- Avoid jackets and tops with extra padding as they'll just make you look bulkier.

- Steer clear of shapeless, bulky jumpers for the same reason.

- If you've got a big belly, go for trousers and a jacket in the same colour to streamline. Single-breasted jackets are more slimming than double-breasted.

- Buy the right size! Anything clinging over a large belly looks slobby.

'Looking stylish is not about following fashion, losing weight, being rich or succumbing to the knife. It's about dressing to show off what you love and hiding what you loathe about your body.'
TRINNY WOODALL and SUSANNAH CONSTANTINE, *What Not To Wear*

- Dark coloured jeans are more flattering than light denim ones.

- Beware of heels for men. Cowboy boots or shoes with a built-in heel won't make you long taller and leaner, they'll just make you look silly and sad.

- Shirts with a vertical stripe will make you look slimmer, as will a tie that is simple and predominantly one colour. Cartoon ties and mad prints are best worn by the very young.

- Go for looser fits and ensure that you can do your trousers up somewhere near your waist.

- Choose fine knits that skim the body. A v neck lengthens, and is especially good if you have a large neck. A polo neck can make you look square-shaped.

Q Are there any rules about handbags?

A Little fussy bags may be cute, but can look silly on a larger frame. If you need to take a small one out in the evening, keep it chic, simple and one colour. An oversized bag doesn't do much for creating a longer, leaner silhouette, especially if the weight of it has you leaning to one side just to walk along the street. If you're large-busted, it will just add to the top-heavy look. A medium-sized bag that is colour-coordinated with what you're wearing is the way to go.

Q What about all the shaping underwear you can buy. Is it worth spending the money?

A Yes it is and there's a lot to choose from, from bras that minimise the bust to pants and tights that trim the tummy, bottom and thighs. Just make sure you buy them in the right size to start with, otherwise they'll create rolls of flab outside the garment!

Q What about jewellery?

A Keep it small and neat to distract the eye. A big choker necklace, for example, will emphasise a chubby neck, just as a chunky bracelet will cover, rather than show off, a slim wrist. For men, a nice chunky watch works better on big hands and wrists than on small ones.

How did it go?

169

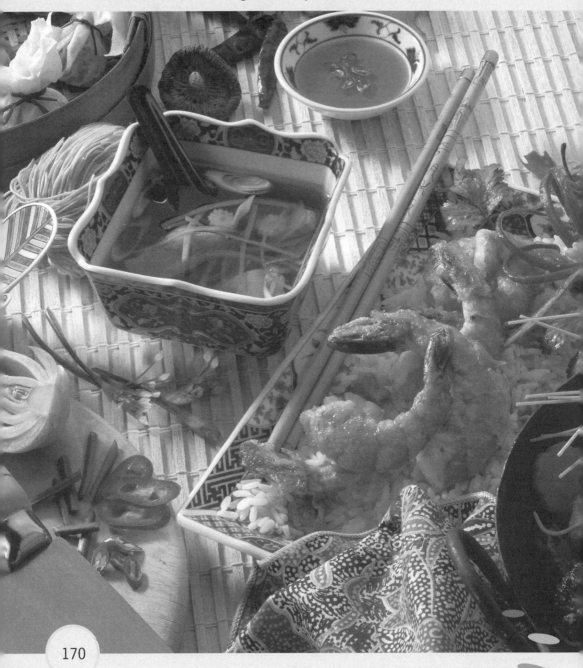

39

I can't eat that because my allergy means it'll pile on pounds

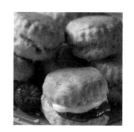

Food allergies and intolerances are very real. They can be fatal. But can they make you fat or is it just a fashionable excuse?

Lots of people latch on to the latest fad in allergies to justify their poor eating habits, which does not do them, or the genuine sufferers, any favours.

Years ago I had a raft of food allergy tests because it was the late 80s and it was 'in' to blame weight gain on certain foods. Apparently if I gave up courgettes I would lose that extra half stone I wanted to shift. Give them up? We were barely on first name terms! It was a waste of time and money. Years later, via my daughter, I came to understand real food allergies. She's allergic to peanuts, as are increasing numbers of people these days, and that's not fun. In fact, it can be fatal. So what are allergies and intolerances all about and how do they affect us?

Here's an idea for you...

In a study on laughter, one group sat quietly in a room while another group watched a stand-up comic. Blood samples taken later showed that the group who had been laughing had a significant increase in their immune system boosters, such as T-lymphocytes, and reduced cortisol, the stress hormone.

A proper food allergy occurs when your body responds to a substance with an immunological reaction. That is, it releases histamine and other chemicals into your blood stream to fight the invader. It may make your skin itch, cause hives or an asthma attack. It can also lead to changes in the blood vessels and swelling of the tongue and throat. The most severe reaction is anaphylactic shock, in which you're struggling for breath and could die. Avoidance of the allergen is the best course of action. Sufferers also get used to carrying an adrenaline injection pen with them.

Food intolerances don't involve an immunological reaction, but can still be unpleasant. They include enzyme defects. For example, a lactose deficiency makes you unable to digest lactose, the milk sugar, and can cause various bowel problems and migraines. You can also suffer pharmacological reactions in response to various components of food, such as amines in coffee and chocolate. Other foods can have an irritant effect, causing quite alarming symptoms such as palpitations and chest pains. A reaction to monosodium glutamate used in Chinese restaurant food can do this – and make you think you're having a heart attack! Food intolerances can be difficult to pin down, too. Your symptoms can be anything from migraines to anxiety, to aching muscles or water retention. You know there's something wrong, but nine times out of ten your doctor will say you just have to live with it.

Defining idea...

'I'm allergic to food. Every time I eat it, I break out in fat.'
JENNIFER GREENE DUNCAN

With all of these, it's essential to be properly diagnosed by a doctor or nutritionist who can do various sensitivity tests and help you with a food elimination diet where you cut out what you think you could be sensitive to and gradually reintroduce it, watching for a reaction.

Stuck on that last half a stone? Check out the ten-point plan in IDEA 49, *Stuck on those last 7 lb.*

Try another idea...

All of these issues are very real, but various diet gurus and alternative health practitioners jump on the food intolerance bandwagon and say if you only give up X and Y, you'll not only feel fantastic, but drop loads of excess weight into the bargain. Not true! It is hard to lose weight. It takes time, discipline and lifestyle changes. The desire to lose weight also makes you vulnerable to quackery; how reassuring it is to be told that your weight problem has nothing to do with anything except your intolerance to, say, wheat or dairy products.

These unscrupulous types often base their spurious claims on wheat and dairy products, because intolerance to these foods is relatively common. Dairy products can be a problem if you're lactose-intolerant, for example. Wheat can also be an issue, but you would probably be diagnosed by a conventional doctor as having coeliac disease, which is when your body reacts to gluten, a constituent of wheat. Symptoms include extreme tiredness, abdominal pains, aching joints, moodiness, migraine, asthma and a stuffy nose. Coeliac disease prevents you from absorbing nutrients properly, resulting in

'Given that the most common sources of food intolerance are wheat and milk, such therapists can achieve a reasonable success rate by diagnosing sensitivity to these two foods in all their patients.'
JONATHAN BROSTOFF, *The Complete Guide to Food Allergy and Intolerance*

Defining idea...

various deficiencies and weight loss, and you have to follow a wheat-free diet more or less permanently.

The upshot is that while you could have an intolerance to foods, diagnosis is difficult because of the wide variety of symptoms. Don't let anyone hoodwink you into thinking you have an intolerance which means you can't lose or stop gaining weight. You'll just end up spending a lot of money without getting the results you deserve, like me and my courgettes. See an allergy specialist or nutritionist to rule out anything serious and then concentrate on tried and tested methods of weight loss.

How did it go?

Q   **Crikey, what can you eat if you can't eat wheat?**

A   *If you're told you have to go on a gluten-free or wheat-free diet, it can be terrifying at first. You have to read food labels very carefully; even stock cubes can contain wheat flour, for example. You'll find that plenty of shops now stock special gluten free ranges however, and it is fine to eat rice, buckwheat (despite the name, it's not wheat), millet, corn, potato flour, and many more flours and grains. Arm yourself with a good wheat-free cookbook.*

Q   **Aren't there pills you can take if you are lactose intolerant?**

A   *You can eat a more varied diet if you use lactose replacers that help digest the lactose if taken at the same time as milky food. They are quite widely available. It is worth trying different brands to see which works best for you.*

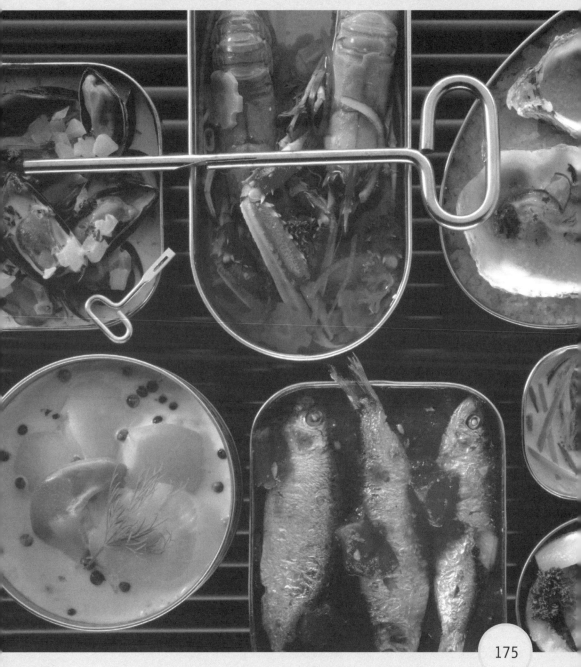

175

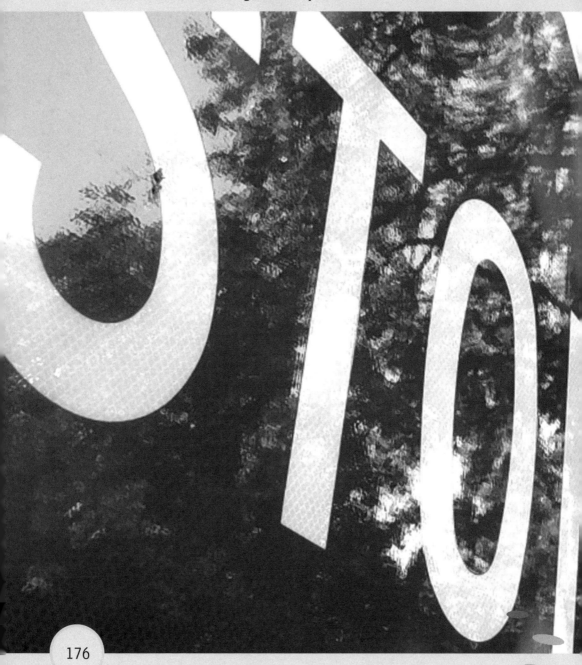

40

Trust me, I'm a doctor

The Atkins diet and other low carbohydrate/high protein diets are in fashion, but they are as controversial as they are popular. Would eating this way work for you, and is it safe?

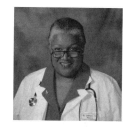

You can't open a magazine or a newspaper these days without seeing some reference to the late Dr Atkins and his amazing diet. His ideas have reached millions through his books.

I know lots of people who swear by his methods and say their lives have been changed, but there are many doctors, nutritionists and other health professionals who have rubbished his views. Others have taken his ideas and refined them. Atkins maintains that traditional low-fat diet recommendations have led to diets high in carbohydrate instead, which are all wrong for our metabolisms. He also says that fat isn't the baddie it is made out to be – at least, not all fats. Is this a case of the mainstream being slow to catch on? After all, Atkins pointed out that it took us centuries to accept that the world was not flat!

Try a carb curfew. Pioneered by British health and fitness expert Joanna Hall, the rule is to eat no carbs after five o'clock. It's a neat way to avoid excess carbohydrates, cuts some calories, and you don't go to bed feeling bloated.

It is beyond the scope of this chapter to go into all his ideas in detail, but let's look at some of the main premises:

THE ATKINS THEORY

We should be concentrating our efforts on our insulin levels, which control sugar levels in the body and how the body stores fat. If you eat a lot of carbohydrates, insulin is released which encourages the body to store the energy from food as fat. You can be 'insulin resistant', which means your body releases very high levels of insulin just to maintain normal blood sugar levels, encouraging more fat to be stored.

Switching to low levels of carbohydrate intake leads your body to burn fat as its energy source, rather than glucose from carbohydrates. Eating fat doesn't affect your blood sugar and, contrary to popular opinion, can be good for your health. Fat also helps you to feel satisfied after eating.

'The perfect diet for those who love food.'
NIGELLA LAWSON

IN PRACTICE

The Atkins diet requires you to start on an induction plan that lasts a minimum of fourteen days. It's pretty strict, including rules such as eating no more than 20 g of carbohydrates a day, which should come from salad greens and certain other 'acceptable' vegetables; no fruit, bread, grains or dairy foods other than cheese, cream and butter; plenty of poultry, fish and meat; no caffeine, processed foods and refined sugars. As you progress, you move through another three phases, culminating in your lifetime maintenance plan. Each phase changes what you can and can't eat; for instance, later on you eat less fat than in the beginning.

Read up on another eating formula that gets the thumbs up from many experts. Turn to IDEA 43, *What's the next big thing?*

Try another idea...

You have to follow the diet to the letter or it won't work, and it's not for the short term – it's a way of eating for life.

WHAT'S THE VERDICT?

Critics have raised concerns about high fat intakes because of the risk of heart disease, but there are studies that show that the diet can have a beneficial effect on cholesterol levels and fats in the blood in the longer term. Kidney damage is another charge levelled at the diet, but there's no real proof. Atkins makes it clear that the diet is not for those who have kidney disease, or for pregnant women and nursing mothers. If you're diabetic, speak to your doctor about the diet. Diabetics can follow the Atkins diet, but only under very careful medical supervision.

Would I recommend it? Despite the fact that it flies in the face of most mainstream thinking, if you're fit and healthy, give it a try. It's down to personal experience in the end, and whether you can stick to it. I couldn't, although I still try to keep my carbohydrate intake controlled. I have also noticed that men seem to get on better with it than women. It must be the lure of all that meat!

'Atkins has never been about no carbs. It's about choosing the right carbs in the right amount.'
Dr STUART TRAGER, Medical Director of Atkins Nutritionals Inc.

Defining idea...

How did it go?

Q **Is it true that you get constipation and smelly breath doing the Atkins diet?**

A *Yes, some people do get constipated, particularly in the early stages. You should drink plenty of water, which should help. Atkins suggests taking a tablespoon of psyllium husks, coarse wheat bran or flaxseed meal each day. The breath thing is to do with ketones, which are fat breakdown chemicals and most common in the induction phase. Some perceive it as odd, sweetish smelling breath, others as horrid. Water, chewing parsley and frequent teeth-cleaning should sort it out.*

Q **What about all the health benefits of fruit and vegetables? We're always being told to eat more, but here you're not allowed them.**

A *Dr Atkins isn't against fruit and veg at all. There are restrictions during the first phase, but plenty of fruit and vegetables are allowed thereafter. He's not too keen on starchy ones, such as sweet potatoes, peas and corn. He thoroughly approves of berries.*

Q **What happens if I have a massive carb binge?**

A *You will get sent straight to the head teacher's office for punishment! If you do have a binge, you just have to go back to the strict induction regime for a few days. And sit in detention by yourself, writing lists of the carbohydrate contents of various foods...*

41

Does being overweight really matter?

Perhaps you never got back into shape after having kids or maybe you've always been a little plumper than you would like. How do you know if it's really a problem?

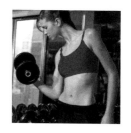

A very attractive, curvaceous woman in her early sixties once said to me, 'Eve, darling, don't ever get too thin, it's so ageing.' And she was right!

I have friends who are in their early thirties and are incredibly proud of their skinny little size 8 or 10 frames, but look at least ten years older with their dried-up faces and flat little bottoms. I think a few curves and a couple of extra kilos are flattering and sensual – and that goes for men too.

When does a little plumpness become unacceptable? It depends on your viewpoint. If carrying a *few* extra kilos doesn't bother you, then it is not an issue. If it annoys you because you want to be in better shape, or it diminishes your confidence or stops you wearing the clothes you want to wear, then you should do something about it. If you have more than a few extra kilos, it does start to matter and when you're properly overweight it starts to matter very much indeed.

Get out your tape measure and calculator. Divide your waist measurement by your hip measurement (in centimetres). If the result is more than 0.95 for a man or 0.87 for a woman, you are apple-shaped. If you are apple-shaped, with more fat around your middle, your risk of heart disease is greater than if you're pear-shaped, with more fat on your bottom.

Fatness is a worldwide epidemic. In the UK alone, it is estimated that two-thirds of men and half of women are overweight, with one in five being obese, that is at least 12.5 kg (28 lb) overweight. Experts are predicting that one in four adults will be obese by 2010.

Obesity makes everyday life uncomfortable is so many ways, such as being unable to run for a bus, a lack of choice in clothes, rude stares and comments from other, thinner, people, and sleep and fertility problems. It is also the commonest cause of ill health and potentially fatal diseases. Obesity contributes to heart disease, diabetes, gallstones and some cancers. Just being overweight – and that's more than say a kilo or so – can raise your blood pressure and give you problems with cholesterol. Even dental decay is more common in overweight people.

In case you're in any doubt as to why being overweight does matter, here are some fat facts to consider:

According to the British Heart Foundation, heart and circulatory disease is the UK's biggest killer. Although the numbers are in fact slightly lower than twenty years ago, this is because of medical advances, not because we are getting healthier! There are other risk factors too, such as smoking, poor psychological health and inherited infirmities, but the truth is that 30% of deaths from coronary heart disease are directly linked to an unhealthy diet. The World Health Organisation estimates that somewhere between 1 and 24% of coronary heart disease is due to doing less than two and a half hours of moderate activity a week.

For another good health reason to get yourself in shape, see IDEA 45, *Could you have diabetes?*

Try another idea...

The fatter you are, the greater your risk. A weight gain of just 10 kg doubles your risk of heart disease. Reducing your weight even by 5 or 10% can have a beneficial effect on cholesterol levels.

Excess weight plays a part in high blood pressure, which can lead to blood clots, stroke and heart attacks. You can reduce these risks through diet: less salt, lower fat consumption and a huge increase in fruit and vegetable consumption.

Although the exact relationships are not fully understood, diet and cancer have an association too. A recent report suggested that as many as 40% of cancers have a dietary link. Breast cancer risk rises with a high fat diet or being overweight.

Clearly there's still a lot of research to be done, but it is certain that being overweight isn't fun and it isn't clever – and it can be about a lot more than the way you look.

'Imprisoned in every fat man a thin one is wildly signalling to be let out.'
CYRIL CONNOLLY

Defining idea...

183

How did
it go?

Q   **I smoke and know I should give up, but I'm already overweight. I don't want to put on even more weight, which always happens when you quit. What shall I do?**

A   *Lots of people find that they put on up to 5 kg (10 lb) when they give up smoking. It's thought that nicotine somehow increases the metabolic rate. When you stop it lowers, which means if you eat the same amount, you will gain weight. Also when you first stop, you can't help snacking more (often out of boredom). This does tend to even out over a period of months. One way to keep weight gain down is to up your activity levels – as much as for distraction as burning up energy! Ultimately the benefits of not smoking have to be worth it. You could also try talking to your doctor about drugs, such as Zyban, that could help you quit without piling on the pounds.*

Q   **How does diet affect your cholesterol levels?**

A   *Firstly cholesterol isn't all bad, in fact it's needed by the body, but it's about the levels of the two kinds of cholesterol. HDL cholesterol is the good stuff, but LDL is the one you want less of. Trans fats (when liquid oils are hardened by hydrogenation in the manufacturing process) and saturated fats (found in meat, cream, butter, full fat milk and so on) cause LDL to rise, while fibre, vegetables and poly- and monounsaturated fats (think olive oil, sunflower oil and fish oils) not only lower LDL, but also boost levels of HDL cholesterol.*

42

The birds and the bees

There's a lot to be said for putting some loving into slimming. Oh come on, don't be shy, everyone does it, you know. Let's talk about sexercise.

Not all the good things in life are bad for you, although it often seems that way when you're trying to lose weight. Sex is definitely slimming.

Although you might be thinking you'd prefer a family-sized bar of fruit and nut chocolate to sex, or just a nice cup of tea, as Boy George once said, it's time to start thinking of love and sex as powerful weapons in your weight-loss armoury. How so? Being in love inspires you like nothing else. You look and feel great, feel happy and full of confidence. It's a great base to start your weight loss plan from because you feel so motivated. And sex? It burns calories, should make you feel good, oh and so much more. So, let's slip into something more comfortable, put some romantic music on the stereo and have a grown up chat.

Here's an idea for you... **Try a sensual aromatherapy massage to get you both in a loving mood. Just add five drops of your chosen essential oil to 20 ml of a carrier oil, such as almond or sunflower. Lavender, rose and camomile are all good relaxers. If you throw in a few drops of juniper or cypress that's supposed to be good for cellulite too!**

LOVE AND SEX LESSON 1

Sex is a great booster for your self-esteem. Despite the fact that if you're trying to lose weight you might feel self-conscious about the way you look, learning to let yourself go is important for intimacy. Besides, virtually all research shows that men have no idea what cellulite is and that women go for personality, not looks (well, maybe they go for looks second). The key is to try to stop dwelling on what you don't like about your body. And when your partner compliments you, even if it is only about your ears, accept it, believe it and enjoy it. If you feel more comfortable with the lights out, turn those lights out or light a few candles, which makes everyone look like Richard Burton and Elizabeth Taylor, Brad and Jen, or Shrek and Princess Fiona. Oh, you know what I mean. It makes everyone look good. And if you feel the need for some covering, a sexy negligee, corset or nurses outfit won't fail to impress. Chaps, there's nothing sexier than you just out of the shower wearing a clean white towel wrapped around your middle, your hair slightly wet, your body lightly oiled, a faint hint of Eau Sauvage…gosh, I'm getting quite carried away.

Defining idea... **'I'd like to meet the man who invented sex and see what he's working on now.'**
ANONYMOUS

LOVE AND SEX LESSON 2

Sex helps you win the battle of the bulge. According to a study in the US, if you make love three times week, you'll burn approximately 7,500 calories a year, which is the same as jogging 120 km (75 miles). Not bad, eh? Of course you do have to actively participate, as opposed to lying there wondering what you're going to eat tomorrow, but still, even kissing burns a few calories a minute. Sex also releases endorphins, those feel-good chemicals that you get after exercising, plus it relaxes you, which is useful as there's a definite link between stress and heart disease as well as weight gain.

If that's got you going, rev yourself up even more with IDEA 16, *Metabolism masterclass.*

Try another idea...

LOVE AND SEX LESSON 3

Sex helps you to sleep, which is a good thing as long as it's not in the middle of a love session. Lack of sleep has been shown to increase snacking and the urge for high-calorie quick energy foods.

LOVE AND SEX LESSON 4

Sex makes you look younger and helps you stay healthy. All that stress reduction and the increased blood supply that you get with regular love-making makes you look more youthful. It boosts your immune system and could help to reduce cholesterol levels. The younger you feel, the more you'll feel like having sex. And of course, sex is a way of strengthening your relationship, of feeling cared for, cherished and respected, which boosts your self-esteem, which means that anything is possible, including losing weight. See, it's all connected.

'Being deeply loved by someone gives you strength, while loving someone deeply gives you courage.'
LAO TZU

Defining idea...

How did it go?

Q **We're so busy, we don't have time for romance. What can we do?**

A *Try something out of the ordinary to get away from ordinary everyday life. Book into a B&B for a night, have a sexy finger food picnic by candlelight in the garden or in front of the fire, take a day off work and go to the countryside or the beach and walk, or chat about anything as long as it's not domestic stuff or work-related. Take the time to really listen to your partner too, even if you think you have heard the jokes and moans a million times before.*

Q **What aphrodisiac foods are there that won't blow my diet?**

A *The aroma of almonds is said to induce passion in women. It's OK to eat a few as well. Chickpeas were fed to stallions by the Romans for mating purposes and they were thought to work well on men too. A sprinkle of nutmeg on your food might be worth a try – it's been prized as an aphrodisiac by Chinese women for centuries. Ginger, chillis, cinnamon and cloves are also said to boost blood flow and make you sweat slightly, two things that could heighten feelings of arousal – or just make you want to step outside for a breath of cool air. Lean steak is rich in B vitamins, zinc and iron, which can all affect sex hormones and the libido. And then there are always oysters, which are full of zinc. Even the act of swallowing them can be very erotic.*

43

What's the next big thing?

Heard about the glycaemic index? If you've been left feeling confused, not to mention hungry and still overweight by other diets, perhaps the GI diet or one of its relatives could be the one for you.

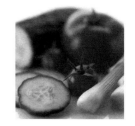

Celebrity fans of the glycaemic index (GI) way of eating are rumoured to include Kylie Minogue. If it could give you a bottom like hers, you'd be mad to not give it a whirl, wouldn't you?

I've got lots of time for this kind of diet because it's easy to follow and live with. It works for vegetarians, too. The GI diet is basically pretty healthy and I've seen people achieve great results with it. So what's it about?

Originally developed during research for diabetes, the glycaemic index is a measure of how quickly you digest various foods and convert them into your body's energy source: glucose. Glucose, or sugar is rated at 100 and everything else gets scored against that. So cornflakes come in at 84, for example, while oatmeal is 42.

Here's an idea for you... **Next time you are shopping, see if you can find GI information on the food label. As well as the full GI listings and information that is available in specialist books, some forward-thinking supermarkets are starting to label products with a low GI and medium GI rating.**

Eating low GI foods means you're satisfied for longer, while those with high ratings on the index not only make you feel hungry again quicker (cue snacking), but also trigger off various processes that lead to fat formation and fat storage. However, that's not the whole picture. The GI diet, to take one of my favourites (by Rick Gallop) also promotes eating a combination of low GI foods that are low in sugar and fat, therefore calories too. Foods are rated red light – avoid, amber – eat occasionally and green – as much as you want. Is this starting to make sense?

The GI diet also recommends playing with balance of your plate, which is not a circus trick, but still a clever kind of juggling. It means creating a mix on your plate that is a little different to mainstream healthy eating guidelines, of 50% vegetables, with another 25 per cent of meat or fish and the remaining 25% rice, pasta or potatoes. As far as serving sizes go, moderation and common sense are encouraged, but suggestions such as 100 g (4 ounces) of meat and 40 g (1.5 ounces) of dry weight pasta are given. Fruit and vegetables tend to be unlimited, though they have to be the green-lighted ones. For instance, boiled new potatoes are 56 on the index, while a baked potato is 84.

What might your breakfast look like on the GI diet? Here's a taster:

- You could have fresh fruit, although not all fruits are green-lighted. Melon for example is out as it's quickly digested. As juice is processed and therefore digested more quickly, whole fruits are better.

- Porridge and sugar-free bran cereals are allowed, as is wholemeal bread that is labelled stoneground – this means less of the fibre is separated, i.e. it'll take longer to digest. A bread serving is one slice and to be eaten sparingly.

- You can have skimmed milk and low or no-fat yoghurts, with artificial sweeteners to keep the calories down.

- No butter is allowed, so you have to shop for non-hydrogenated soft margarine.

- Spreads such as reduced sugar or sugar-free jams are fine.

What are the secrets of successfully maintaining your weight loss? As well as a healthful diet, there are other tricks you need to know to IDEA 52, *Zen and the art of weight loss maintenance.*

Try another idea...

191

'I decided to try this diet. To my amazement and delight I lost the twenty pounds that had been plaguing me for so long.'
RICK GALLOP, author of the *GI Diet*

What you can't have are sausages and regular bacon (a bit of leaner back bacon or lean ham is fine), full fat dairy products, white refined produce, such as baguettes, muffins and croissants and dried fruit or fruits that are canned in syrup. My only real gripe as far as the breakfast goes is that coffee isn't allowed – well, only the decaffeinated sort. This is due to caffeine increasing insulin production and reducing blood sugar levels, which makes you hungry.

Overall, the diet is supposed to be a way of eating for life, rather than using as a short-term diet. As it's healthy and easy to follow, that doesn't present a problem. Yes, there are things you have to cut out, some temporarily and some long term, but in truth, they're things that ultimately don't do you health or weight any good anyway. The diet also endorses exercise – an essential in my book! So, yes, this one gets the green light from me.

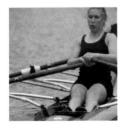
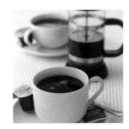
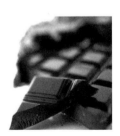

Q   How long will it take me to lose weight on the GI diet?

A   *The first phase is supposed to take between three and six months based on a 10% reduction in your weight. Although this might sound quite a long time, it does mean that you're losing weight at a safe rate, as opposed to losing lots at once and then plateauing. Besides, it's not really that long in terms of the rest of your life. If we can really establish a life-long habit of healthy eating and exercise, we may never have to diet again. Wouldn't that be wonderful?*

Q   Are there variants of the GI eating plan, just like there are variants of the high protein/low carbohydrate diets?

A   *Yes there are and they all have subtle differences, though using the index as the basis for their recommendations. There is also a plethora of GI cookbooks – a worthwhile investment if you like the sound of eating this way.*

Q   What does the GI diet say about chocolate and alcohol?

A   *They are strictly forbidden! No, just kidding. You are allowed the occasional bit of chocolate, as long it's one of those with a high cocoa content, which usually have less fat and sugar than regular chocolate. Alcohol is allowed after you've done the first phase of the diet, but always only in moderation.*

How did it go?

193

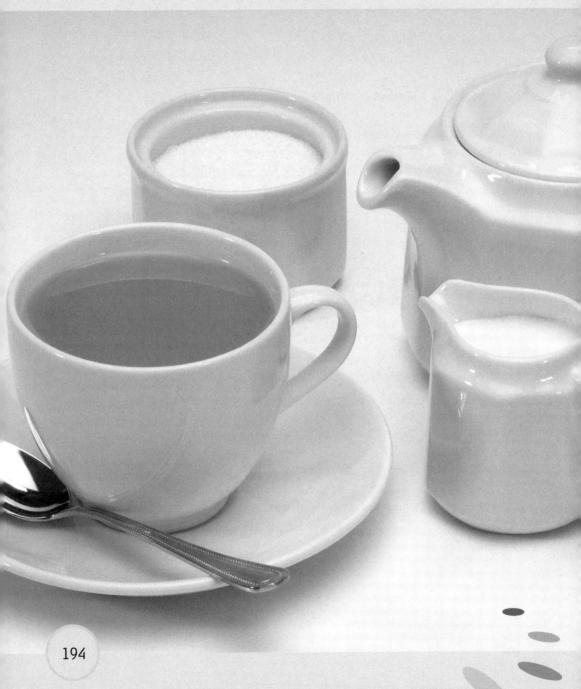

44

Time for tea (would you like black, green, herbal or slimming?)

It's a seductive idea: sip tea and watch the weight melt away. But can a tea ever really be more than a refreshing drink?

Let me read your tea leaves. I see a large shape saying this cup of diet tea was a waste of time. Stick to sensible eating and more exercise instead of lying around drinking your brew of 'Bye Bye Fat'.

We all like an easy option, and what could be easier than sipping yourself slim with a fat-busting tea? Health food stores offer some of these super-charged brews, but it's on the internet that you're really spoiled for choice. And it's also on the internet that you can say or sell just about anything you want and get away with it. As with many things in life, not all everything is what it seems, and tea is no exception.

Here's an idea for you...

Make your own herbal tea or infusion. Use a teaspoon of dried herbs or two of fresh to a cup of boiling water. Pour the water over the herbs and leave it covered for five to ten minutes. Before you drink it, strain it.

Let's take black tea, which is the regular tea you find everywhere, and green tea first of all. Both contain flavonoids with myriad health benefits including protection against heart disease. This is proven, so drink up and you'll do yourself some good. Just use skimmed milk and limit the sugar. Green tea has been in the spotlight recently, following various research projects. It has been linked with having a preventative effect on all kinds of diseases, including certain cancers, as well as having the ability to lower cholesterol and, to speed up fat oxidation, i.e. to burn calories quicker. Further research is needed in all these areas, but it's safe to say that if you like the taste of green tea, you've got nothing to lose apart from just possibly a few kilos.

TRIED AND TRUSTED?

Herbal teas go back a long way and are used in both traditional Chinese and Indian medicine. They're popular everywhere as an alternative to regular tea and coffee and in some countries are used as "cures" for common complaints, including for example, fennel as an aid to digestion and camomile to ease anxiety and promote sleep. Of course quite how healing they are is a matter for debate, primarily because they may not in fact contain enough of the herb to have any effect. But still, a herbal tea whose ingredient you recognise won't do you any harm at all. It's the blends that are given compelling weight-loss promising names that you need to be cautious about.

In fact, many people think diet teas, which contain ingredients such as licorice root, senna and buckthorn, should really be called laxative teas because that's what they do to you! In small amounts they can just be a little, well, inconvenient, as you have to run to the loo rather a lot. If you consume them in large amounts, you're asking for trouble. Others act as diuretics, especially if they have dandelion, parsley or juniper as ingredients, so you lose water weight. Then there are the diet teas that contain stimulants such as yerba mate, kola nut and guarana. They're OK in small doses, but if you're sensitive to the ingredients or have just a little too much, you'll get palpitations, the jitters and have difficulty sleeping. It's rare, but there's a risk of heart attack. Since the only reason you'll be drinking the teas that are marketed as slimming aids is to lose weight (most of them don't actually taste that great) and as there's absolutely no proof that they can help, I'd leave them well alone. Stick to a nice cup of real tea, or traditional herbal tea that doesn't make any other claim than it tastes good!

But aren't there useful supplements and medical diet pills that could work for me? Yes, there are, but they are aids to weight-loss, not substitutes for exercise and a good diet. Turn to IDEA 46, *Couldn't I just pop a pill?*

Try another idea...

'Drinking a daily cup of tea will surely starve the apothecary.'
CHINESE PROVERB

Defining idea...

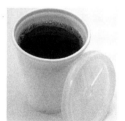

How did
it go?

Q   Doesn't normal tea have caffeine in it, so can't it give you the jitters too?

A   *Yes, tea does contain caffeine, but at far lower levels than coffee, regular cola drinks and chocolate bars. You'd have to drink an awful lot to get twitchy side effects, unless of course you were particularly sensitive.*

Q   It's a diuretic too, isn't it?

A   *According to recent research, no. You'd have to drink five or six cups at one sitting to clock up the 250–300 mg of caffeine needed to create a diuretic effect. In fact, it is now acknowledged that tea can contribute to your daily fluid intake, which is recommended to be 1.5–2 litres a day. In the UK, most people drink on average three to four cups of tea. That might sound like a nice bit of trivia, but it shows that some seemingly old-fashioned habits really aren't so bad after all.*

Q   How should you drink it?

A   *You can drink it hot with milk or lemon or cold with ice. It's up to you. It won't affect the health-giving properties of green or black tea, so drink it the way you like it. Ideally, though, don't drink it with meals, as it decreases the absorption of iron from foods.*

45

Could you have diabetes?

Diabetes is increasing on a global scale. Even more concerning is the fact that you could be a sufferer without knowing it. Here's what is has to do with diet and activity levels

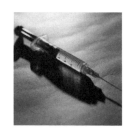

Diabetes is a chronic and incurable disease with nasty complications, such as blindness, kidney failure, stroke and nerve damage.

Diabetes is not new – in the 17th century it was called the 'pissing evil' – but it is on the increase. There are two types of diabetes. Type 1 is more commonly found in children and young adults and is treated with a strict diet and insulin injections. It's Type 2 that is on the increase and is strongly linked to obesity and a lack of activity. There are other risk factors over which we have no control, such as genetic inheritance, simply getting older and your ethnic origin – Asians and Afro-Caribbeans do seem to be at a higher risk. Eating lots of sweet things, contrary to popular belief, doesn't cause diabetes, but it leads to weight gain, which does increase your risk. It's a fact that 80% of people with Type 2 diabetes are overweight. The fatter and less fit you are, the greater your risk.

Here's an idea for you...

How can you get five fruit and vegetables into your daily diet? Try having one piece of fruit at breakfast, plus a piece of fruit after lunch or as an afternoon snack; have a salad with lunch or dinner and two vegetables (not potatoes) with your other meal.

Type 2 diabetes used to be more common in middle age, but increasingly it's affecting younger people too. Those with the condition either don't produce enough insulin or what is produced doesn't work effectively, which means that the body can't use glucose properly and levels remain high in the blood. Some of the symptoms of undiagnosed diabetes include increased thirst, a need to go to the toilet often, especially at night, lethargy and tiredness, blurred vision, regular thrush and genital itching, plus weight loss when nothing else has changed regarding your lifestyle. Doctors say many people have these symptoms on and off for years before eventually being diagnosed as diabetic, which is easily done with a simple blood test.

In the past, if you were diagnosed as having diabetes, physical activity was discouraged and, a high fat/low carbohydrate diet prescribed. How times change! Now exercise is encouraged, just as it is for everyone to improve their health and control weight. As a role model, look to Sir Steve Redgrave, five times Olympic Gold medal winner and a diabetes sufferer! Diet-wise, the reason a high fat diet was recommended was to make up for the lack of calories that resulted from following a low carbohydrate diet to keep sugar levels stable (fat doesn't boost sugar levels in itself). Diabetics are more at risk of heart disease as a result of the condition, but of course, the high fat diet increased this risk! Luckily, nutrition has moved on, with eating guidelines for diabetics pretty much in line with general healthy eating recommendations. As well as using medication and being under strict medical supervision, most diabetics can control their condition and also lose weight by eating in the most healthful way. The eating guidelines also work as a preventative and can be used by everyone. In brief, they are:

IDEA 48, *The incredible bulk*, tells you more about the benefits of unrefined foods, fruits and vegetables.

Try another idea...

■ Eat regular meals featuring starchy carbohydrates of the whole grain variety, i.e. wholemeal bread and cereals, rather than refined carbohydrates.

■ Cut down on fat, especially saturated fats found in animal products. Choose low fat and monounsaturated fats such as olive oil.

■ Eat more fruit and vegetables!

■ Cut down on sugar and sugary foods, especially sugary drinks which cause blood glucose levels to rise quickly.

■ Cut down on salt to keep blood pressure in check and drink in moderation. Diabetics in particular should be careful of drinking on an empty stomach, as it can precipitate hypoglycaemia – dangerously low blood sugar levels.

'According to one recent study on diabetes care conducted in the US, on average for every 1 kg (2 lb) in weight a person puts on over the normal range, their risk of developing diabetes increases by about 9 per cent.'
JUDITH MILLS, *The Diet Bible*

Defining idea...

How did
it go?

Q What about special diabetic foods?

A   *Most experts say they are unnecessary and a waste of money.*

Q Isn't Type 2 diabetes just a mild form of the illness?

A   *No, it needs to be taken seriously. Four out of five people with the condition die prematurely from heart disease. There's also an increased risk of stroke, diabetic vetinopathy which can lead to blindness, and nerve damage in the hands and feet. Action is essential, both if you've already been diagnosed and also as a preventative measure with weight control being an important strategy. Recent research has shown that complications are prevented if blood glucose levels are normalised with Type I diabetes. Most experts believe the same for Type II diabetes too.*

Q Surely it's not that big an issue? What about all the plagues and epidemics?

A   *The World Health Organisation thinks it is a big issue. It is predicting a global epidemic of diabetes, which means that it already is an issue for you and it will definitely be an issue for your children and the ones you might have in the future. Do ask your doctor for a test if any of the risk factors apply to you and also if you have any of the symptoms described above.*

46

Couldn't I just pop a pill?

You would think there would be safe, effective, fat-reducing pill that you could buy at the pharmacy. Some would say it's already here in the form of supplements and certain prescription drugs. So what's the truth?

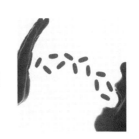

Some years ago when I was editing a health and fitness magazine, we all got very excited about a new fat-busting product that built lean muscle mass. It was a powder that you mixed with water and drank daily — sadly it didn't seem to work.

Eight of us decided to give it go. After a week, seven had given up due to stomach cramps and diarrhoea. The eighth (it was me) carried on. My stomach was fine and I decided I must be quite tough, but at the end of the two month long course I didn't look, weigh or measure any different.

Here's an idea for you...

If you want a herbal appetite suppressant, scientists have now isolated the active molecules in the *Hoodia gordonii* plant, used by tribesmen in the Kalahari to stave off hunger pangs whilst on hunting trips. Some products are already available, being sold as appetite suppressants and anecdotally are getting good reviews. However, more research is needed.

There are many supplements that promise appetite suppression, weight loss and increases in lean muscle mass. These products are widely available through pharmacies, health food stores and of course the good old internet. Often you might find a trainer at your local gym recommending them too. But do any of them actually work? Let's look at a few of the most popular:

Chromium picolinate

Chromium is needed to help insulin transfer glucose and nutrients from the bloodstream to the cells and plays a role in energy production. It's found in foods such as mushrooms and broccoli. The lure of supplements that combine chromium and picolinate is the potential of losing fat and gaining muscle tone – this is based on the results of a number of studies. However, further research hasn't been able to duplicate the original claims and indeed some research has subsequently made links between high levels of supplementation, DNA damage and a host of other nasties. In fact, at time of writing, this substance is facing a ban in the UK.

Chitosan

This is made from crushed crab and lobster shells! The theory is that the fibre from the shells binds with and absorbs the fat from your food before it is metabolised. Some studies have shown it can help weight loss, but there are no large scale convincing trials, so who really knows? The downside is that chitosan will also decrease the absorption of fat-soluble vitamins, plus you'll experience a laxative effect. It is not recommended – especially if you're allergic to shellfish!

Is there any merit in diet teas? Probably not, and they are certainly not a miracle cure. See IDEA 44, *Time for tea*.

Try another idea...

Creatine
Creatine is used by athletes and perhaps a few chaps in your local gym to increase muscular performance. Most studies have been short term. It's not one for average dieters.

Amino acids
These are readily available as pills and powders, but despite the hype there's no proof that they will increase muscle mass or burn fat as a supplement. The only approved use of amino acids is for the intravenous feeding of people with specific health conditions such as kidney disease. You are better off with protein foods such as meat and eggs and plenty of exercise.

DOCTOR'S ORDERS

Producing a weight-control pill is truly one of the Holy Grails of pharmaceutical companies, because anything that even half works is a veritable goldmine. There are already products available. You may have heard of sibutramine, marketed as Reductil, and Orlistat (or Xenical) to name a couple. Trials of a drug called

'*People usually spend more time researching their next car or computer purchase than selecting their supplements.*'
FELICIA BUSCH, *The New Nutrition*

Defining idea...

Rimonabant have also been successful in both weight loss and helping smokers to quit without piling on pounds. At the moment the drugs that are licensed can only be given to you on prescription from your doctor. So what would happen if you went along and asked for your doctor for one of them? As non-pharmacological means of losing weight are still the first line of treatment, you'd probably be sent away with a diet sheet, an appointment with a dietician and advice on getting more physically active. However, if you have a BMI of 30 or more or have been trying without success to lose weight through lifestyle changes, your doctor may well prescribe one of the drugs.

In conclusion, beware of supplements that promise weight loss and muscle tone with no effort. At best they just won't work and will be a waste of money. At worst, they could be dangerous, especially if randomly combined with other supplements and medicines. And if you're not obese, you probably won't be advised to pop a prescription pill. So, it's back to good old fashioned sensible eating and exercise, truly tried and tested and suitable for everyone.

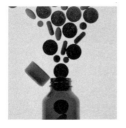 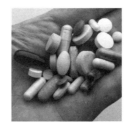 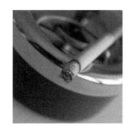

Q   **I thought I'd heard good things about something called leptin. Any truth in them?**

How did it go?

A   *This goes back a few years and relates to some research in rodents in which those with a lack of leptin had increased appetites. The idea was that obese people may be lacking leptin, so if you gave them more, their appetite should reduce. However, leptin is rarely deficient in humans. In fact, obese people can have high levels, though it's mooted that there could be a case for leptin-resistance. The jury is still out. And the researchers are still researching.*

Q   **OK, so if I can't take any pills, how else can I control my appetite?**

A   *Eat little and often to keep your blood sugar levels stable and ward off uncontrollable hunger pangs. Try drinking plenty of fluids to fill you up – anything from water to a bowl of tomato soup. Eat slowly when you have a meal to allow your brain to register more quickly that you are full, and try to sit down rather than eat standing up for the same reason. Avoid sugary snacks that will give you a quick hit, but soon leave you wanting more. Remember to distract yourself from thinking about food. Try doing anything that will take your mind off it!*

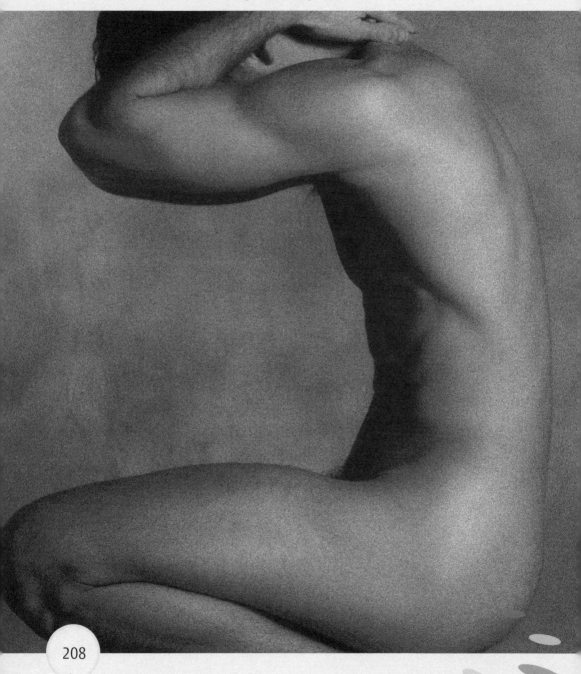

47

Spot reduction: the facts and the fiction

How much can you change your natural shape? Is it possible to lose weight from specific areas of your body? There are many myths surrounding those questions. Here's the truth.

What did you inherit? I don't mean a cottage by the sea or your Great Uncle Stan's stamp collection — I'm talking about things like Mum's thighs and Dad's height.

As well as your gender and your nutrition in childhood, the main influence on your body shape comes from your parents. You can take after one or other of them, or be a mix of both.

Broadly speaking, human shapes can be split into three main types, ectomorphs, mesomorphs and endomorphs. Ectomorphs are tall and thin and are often quite angular or even delicate-looking. They have a low body fat percentage and not

Here's an idea for you...

To get an idea of whether you really need to lose weight or indeed to track your progress, you can have your body fat measured electronically. A harmless electric current is passed through your body which estimates body water, showing the amount of muscle you have. The difference between your overall weight and lean tissue weight gives an idea of your body fat. Gyms and health centres usually offer this service (for a price) or you can also buy special scales to use at home.

much muscle, either. Although they usually have few weight problems when young, they are likely to put on weight around the stomach area as they age. Mesomorphs tend to have quite a bit of muscle and indeed a higher muscle to fat ratio than the other two types. They appear well-built with strong arms and legs. A mesomorph stays in good shape if active. However, a sedentary mesomorph will gain body fat. The endomorph is altogether rounder and softer looking, with more fat than muscle. They put weight on easily, but with regular physical activity can achieve good muscle tone.

As well as the basic shapes, you can have an android or gynoid influence. The android is an apple shape, with most weight carried on the top half of the body (and of course, sooner or later around the abdominal area). This shape is more closely associated with ectomorphs and mesomorphs as they age and especially men, while it affects endomorphs more generally. The gynoid influence, which is a pear shape, i.e. heavier on the bottom half, is a more female shape and can occur across the three groups. While we can be a combination of the groups, most of us do tend to fall into one identifiable type. The key is to identify the closest to your shape and work with it, rather than battling against it, to be in the best possible shape you can be.

MOVERS AND SHAPERS

You cannot spot reduce and lose weight from specific areas of the body. Research has shown that we all tend to lose weight from the top down, so, first it shows in your face, then your chest and stomach area, followed by hips, thighs and legs. Abdominal fat seems to be fairly easy to shift – good news for apple shapes, less good for pear shapes. But of course as abdominal fat is a risk factor in heart disease, pear shaped people can afford to be a little smug. But I'd rather be slim and in proportion, I hear the pear shapes say. A fat pear shaped person will slim into, well, a slimmer pear shaped person. And there's not a lot more you can do about your basic shape apart from surgery, which I don't recommend, but it's up to you. There is also exercise, which I do strongly recommend. One of the best tips for the pear-shaped person is to focus your strength training efforts on your top half to create more balance.

How much can exercise change your shape? Toning exercises certainly work to either increase your muscle bulk or streamline your muscles. However, if you've got lots of fat covering your muscles it will be harder to see muscle definition, plus you could just end up looking bigger. It's best to lose some body fat first. Contrary to popular myth it's not possible to turn fat into muscle or the other way around. Fat is fat and muscle is muscle.

What has sleep got to do with weight control? More than you might think! See IDEA 29, *Snooze and lose.*

Try another idea...

'I'm in shape. Round is a shape, isn't it?'
ANONYMOUS

Defining idea...

211

How did it go?

Q I'm losing weight...and my bust. Can you help?

A *This is a hard one to get around. Just as you can't lose weight from specifically targeted areas, you can't put weight back on selectively either! The best course of action is to do plenty of chest exercises (press ups and the pec dec machine in the gym for example) to work your pectoral muscles around the breast area. While this sort of exercise won't increase the size of your breasts, it will keep them uplifted and perky. Other than that, you can create cleavage using a good push-up bra, one that is filled with gel, or 'chicken fillets', those rubbery shapes to slip inside your bra.*

Q Is there anything I can do to help give a better shape to my waist?

A *Your waist should decease in size as you lose weight overall. Good posture helps too, as do specific Pilates and yoga moves. You can also work your waist with toning exercises that target your oblique muscles that run down the sides of your torso. Talk to a trainer at your local gym or health club and ask to be shown a selection of moves. I have also heard that exercising for ten minutes a day with a hula hoop can whittle inches from your waistline.*

48

The incredible bulk

It comes from plants and cannot be digested, nor does it provide any calories or energy. So what, you may well ask, is the point of fibre? Actually it's fascinating. How long have you got?

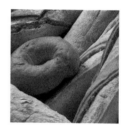

Fibre is about a lot more than chewing on bran flakes to keep you regular. As well as its myriad health benefits, fibre can also help you stay slim.

Generally people with high fibre diets weigh less than those who don't each much fibre. This could be due to the fact that fibre-rich foods are filling. And if you're full you don't feel the need to overeat or snack on treats. A recent paper on weight loss in the US confirmed that low fat diets with plenty of complex carbohydrates, fruit and vegetables are naturally high in fibre and low in calories and as such lead to weight loss. One study even reported that following this kind of eating model, the carbohydrates could be consumed freely and weight would still be lost.

Here's an idea for you...

Drink a litre of juice a day: it's around 400 calories. Drink a litre of water and eat a couple of oranges instead. It will save you calories and give you more fibre. Fruit juice is healthy and full of vitamins and counts as one of five a day fruit and vegetable portions. It's also high in sugars, albeit natural ones.

The benefits of fibre, or to give it its new, proper name, non-starch polysaccharides, have been known for thousands of years. Hippocrates (known as the father of medicine) advised his wealthy patients to follow the example of their servants and eat brown bread rather than white for example, "for its salutary effect on the bowel". Now we now more about fibre itself.

There are two kinds of fibre, soluble and insoluble. They are not nutrients in themselves as they are not digested for the most part, but both have important jobs to do. Soluble fibre lowers blood cholesterol levels and also slows the absorption of glucose into the blood stream ensuring there isn't a sudden rise in blood sugar levels. Although most plant foods combine soluble and insoluble fibre, the former is found particularly in oats and oat bran, barley, brown rice, beans and pulses, and fruit and vegetables. Insoluble fibre keeps things moving along in your digestive system. Look away now if bottom and bowel business makes you feel a little uncomfortable and fidgety. It acts a bit like a sponge and soaks up water to expand the bulk of your waste products (the faeces). Basically with dietary fibre your stools are softer and move along easily, which helps to avoid constipation and piles and also protects against rectal and colon cancers. The best sources of insoluble fibre are wheat, whole grain breads and cereals, corn, green beans and peas and the skins of fruits such as apples.

Defining idea...

'A fruit is a vegetable with looks and money.'
P. J. O'ROURKE

CAN YOU HAVE TOO MUCH OF A GOOD THING?

It's recommended that we eat around 18 g of fibre a day, which most of us barely manage. We don't manage it because we eat more refined carbohydrates (white, processed foods and sugars) and don't eat enough fruit and vegetables. But the benefits are clear to see. When you increase your fibre consumption, make sure you drink plenty of water. You might also find that you retain some fluid at first, making you look and feel a little heavier. And there may be a bit of wind! This is temporary though as you get used to the new foods in your diet. Increasing your activity levels helps as it stimulates the muscles in the torso, helping speedier elimination – you don't want all that waste hanging around. There's some evidence that very high intakes of wheat bran can interfere with the absorption of iron and calcium, but it would need to be consistently high to really cause problems (though it can be a big issue for children and pregnant women). As new research suggests that high fibre consumption from a variety of sources affords a 40 per cent lesser risk of bowel cancer and that women who eat plenty of fruit and vegetables and wholegrain cereals have a lower incidence of breast cancer, it makes sense to increase your dietary fibre and start chewing for health. And of course to keep hunger pangs at bay!

As well as plenty of fibre, you can discover what else a balanced diet should contain in **IDEA 4, *Pyramid selling*.**

Try another idea...

'**There are food scares in Belgium involving everything from poultry to chocolate. To the despair of many worldwide, however, another millennium ends without any bad news about Brussels sprouts.'**
FRANK McNALLY

Defining idea...

215

How did it go?

Q **I've got irritable bowel syndrome and I don't know whether to eat more bran and fibre or whether that will make it worse. Which is it?**

A *A high-fibre diet has always been recommended for IBS, but it doesn't work for everyone. Just as the actual symptoms of IBS can vary, so can the effects of fibre – it can make both diarrhoea and constipation worse for example. Mostly it seems that the problem is with wheat fibre, found in wholemeal bread and often in biscuits and cereal too. The only way to find out if it is this that's making things worse is to cut it out for at least a month, then slowly reintroduce some wholewheat into your diet and see what happens. You'll find you probably won't have problems with refined wheat products, such as white bread and pasta.*

Q **Could I take a fibre supplement?**

A *I wouldn't. Besides there are so many other nutrients in high fibre foods that you'd be missing out on – phytochemicals, minerals and antioxidants that all pack big health benefits.*

Q **Is there any way to avoid the windiness you get after eating pulses?**

A *If you're preparing them yourself, just make sure that they are thoroughly cooked (and, except for lentils and split peas, soaked overnight before cooking). I buy my pulses in cans because I can't be bothered with the lengthy preparation process. Just check they're canned in water only and don't have added sugar or salt. You could also try adding certain herbs to the pulse dishes you're making. Herbs that are claimed to help with wind include thyme, fennel, caraway, rosemary and lemon balm.*

49

Stuck on those last 7lb?

That stubborn half a stone is hard to shift whether you are near the end of your weight loss programme or when 7 lb is all you want to lose to begin with.

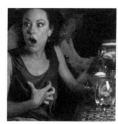

It's such a small amount, you'd think it would pack its bags and leave without a whimper. But no, that half a stone always seems to be trickiest to shift.

I don't know why, but what I do know is that to make it go away you have to re-double your efforts and have more tricks up your sleeve than a magician. Make a start with my ten-point checklist.

1. Be honest with yourself about what you're eating. Keep a food diary for a week and note down everything that you consume. You might think you're eating sensibly, but a diary could help you spot the source of those extra kilos.

2. Do you suffer from portion distortion? Even healthy diet-friendly foods such as fruits have calories. If you eat vast amounts of anything and it exceeds your calorie output, you'll put on weight. Match it and you'll maintain that extra half stone.

Limit your food options: too many choices can make you eat more. Research has shown that volunteers ate 44% more than a control group when offered a variety of dishes rather than the same amount of one dish.

'Habit, if not resisted, soon becomes a necessity.'
ST AUGUSTINE

3. How consistent are you? There are some experts who say as long as you eat sensibly for 80% of the time, you can relax a little for the other 20%. This could translate as making the healthiest choices all week and then eating whatever you like at the weekend. However, there's a big difference between relaxing a little and having a total blow-out every weekend. If you opt for the blow-outs, your week's calorie intake will stack up and your healthful efforts will be for nothing. That dull word 'moderation' springs to mind, but it really is a good concept to live by.

4. Be more active, whatever your current levels of activity, to rev up your rate of weight loss. If you are sedentary start walking or swimming, ideally for at least half an hour five times a week. They are both safe effective exercises that, if done regularly, will pay dividends. If you are reasonably active, or even if you think you work out a lot, try to incorporate some new activities into your week to challenge your mind and body. Try working out for longer, more frequently or harder – or all of these together!

5. A simple way to cut a few calories is to cut out carbohydrates with your evening meal. You could try it every night for a couple of weeks, or every other night if that's more convenient. As long as your other meals and snacks are nutrionally balanced with some carbohydrate, you won't be missing out and you'll definitely see a difference of the scales.

6. Have healthy snacks. If you eat regular well-balanced meals and have a few in-between snacks that are also healthy – not a packet of crisps or bar of chocolate – your blood sugar levels will remain stable and you won't ever feel ravenously hungry, so you're less likely to binge or overeat.

Could alcohol be contributing excess calories? Check out IDEA 32, High spirits

Try another idea...

7. Spice up your life with a few hot peppers in your lunch or dinner. Pepper eaters have less of an appetite and feel full quicker according to Canadian research. The compound capsaicin that is found in peppers temporarily speeds your metabolism.

8. Include calcium in your diet, as, along with other substances in dairy foods, it seems to help your body burn excess fat faster. In a study, women who ate low fat yoghurt and cheese and drank low fat milk three or four times in a day lost 70% more body fat than women who didn't eat dairy at all.

9. Get your rest. Sleep deprivation and a stressed out lifestyle can boost levels of cortisol in your body, which is associated with higher levels of insulin and fat storage. We can interpret the body's cues for sleep as hunger and end up snacking or drinking gallons of coffee to stay awake...and then not be able to sleep.

10. Don't eat when you're not hungry. It seems obvious, but think about it next time you put your food in your mouth. Ask yourself "Am I really hungry?" before that second mouthful.

'It's OK to let yourself go, just as long as you let yourself back.'
MICK JAGGER

Defining idea...

219

How did it go? **Q   Are there some quick-fix beauty treatments that would help shed a few kilos?**

A   Yes, but they'll only help you lose inches by losing water, so won't have anything more than a temporary effect. Still, if you need a boost, I think they're great. Look out for the Universal Contour Wrap, Ionithermie and Shape Changers Detox Wrap Mini Home Kit. Looking after your body and nurturing it, even just by say massaging in body lotion, is a psychologically healthy thing to do. It indicates that you're not at war with your body, which is a positive attitude for diet success.

Q   Should I cut out all fat to speed up my weight loss?

A   No! A moderate consumption of fat gives you taste and variety and besides, we need fats for health. You do need to choose your fats wisely though. They are all calorific, but some bring health benefits to the party too. Trans fats should be avoided as far as possible and you should also try to cut down on saturated fats. Plant oils, oily fish, nuts and avocados are all packed with the beneficial fats that protect against heart disease and other diseases and conditions, so when you do eat fat, choose those.

50

What's your excuse?

We all have them – perfectly good reasons why our diet has failed, where it went wrong, why we can't exercise and so on. Only they're not reasons, they're excuses. Let's expose them one by one.

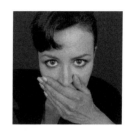

It's my glands! It's my knees! It's because I have to wait for a phone call from my granny to let me know if she needs a lift to the hairdresser's.

Whether they are plausible reasons or fictional tales worthy of Hollywood's finest, the trouble with excuses is that they are stopping you from achieving your goals. Usually there are some powerful emotions struggling underneath these excuses. If you can unravel what they are, it could help you to move on. For example, you may be fearful of failing or of loooking silly. Maybe there's anger inside you, manifesting itself as "I have too many commitments to others to make time for myself". If you can get to the root of negative emotions, you can develop strategies to deal with them. Here's a selection of the excuses we've all heard (and used?!) a million times before, with ideas on how to overcome them:

Eating carbohydrates before you exercise can reduce the amount of fat you burn for hours afterwards. Instead, researchers recommend having a high protein snack, such as a handful of nuts, before your workout.

'I don't have time to exercise.'

This is the commonest excuse that people give for avoiding physical activity. But ask yourself if your life is really that different to people who do exercise. How do they manage? It's so important to exercise both from a weight loss and fitness point of view that you really should try to give it priority. So, if it's childcare that's an issue, could your partner watch the kids, a neighbour or perhaps a fellow mum would be willing to barter babysitting hours with you? Many health clubs also offer crèches. Perhaps you could get up earlier or work out at lunchtime? You don't have to do all your exercise at once either – you could split it into smaller chunks throughout the day.

'Everyone puts on weight as they get older.'

It's not inevitable, unless you consistently overeat whilst being inactive.

'I never had a weight problem until I had children.'

Well give them back then! No, just kidding. Baby weight is lost through sensible eating and physical activity, but you also need to look at your habits. Do you eat up the kids' leftovers or snack constantly because you're so busy rushing around that you don't make time to prepare yourself a nourishing meal? Do you eat with the kids and then later with your partner too? Do you treat yourself at the end of day when kids are packed off to bed with a few glasses of wine or tub of ice-cream?

Defining idea...

'The only way to get rid of a temptation is to yield to it.'
OSCAR WILDE

'I don't feel like exercising.'

If you need motivation, make a commitment to working out with a friend or group. It's hard to let the side down, even if you feel OK about letting yourself down. If you don't feel like it because you don't like exercise, what have you tried? Just because you may not fancy the gym with all its machinery, doesn't mean you wouldn't enjoy classes, sports, swimming or walking. You might love dancing for example, so make a workout out of it by joining a salsa club or even just dancing to all your favourite music in your living room.

If you've ever considered cosmetic surgery as an answer to weight loss, read IDEA 34, *Suck it out*, first.

Try another idea...

'Exercise hurts!'

If it hurts so much you hate it, get dizzy or exhausted, stop. However, if you simply feel some muscle soreness afterwards, it is normal – assuming you warmed up, cooled down and didn't actually injure yourself. The key is not to overdo things, especially if you're new to exercise and have been very sedentary, both to not put yourself off for good and also to avoid injury. Little and often is a good beginning. As you get fitter – and you'll see results in a few weeks – you can push yourself harder.

'I just end up bingeing on all the foods I can't have.'

Well don't deny yourself anything. Have a small amount of your craved food stuff as soon as you want it. Just make sure it is a small amount and then go and do something else. Denial is a recipe for weight gain.

'People are always blaming circumstances for what they are. I do not believe in circumstances. The people who get on in this world are the people who get up and look for the circumstances they want, and if they cannot find them, make them.'
GEORGE BERNARD SHAW

Defining idea...

223

How did
it go?

Q **I'm a morning person, but when is the best time to exercise?**

A *When you feel motivated, I'd say! Research on athletes has shown that the best time for training is actually in the evening, as this is when flexibility, heart rate and body temperature are at their peak. Of course, if you exercise too late, you'll probably be too full of energy to get to sleep for a while. Ultimately, to keep it up, exercise has to fit in to your lifestyle, so whether that means you do it in the morning, at lunchtime or in the evening, it is entirely up to you. The benefits of exercising every day, or most days, are much greater than the time of day at which you do it – so don't use the idea that you have missed the right time of day as an excuse not to exercise!*

Q **Couldn't there be something wrong with my glands?**

A *It's just possible that you have thyroid problems. The symptoms of hypothyroidism, when not enough of the hormone thyroxine is produced, include weight gain, feeling tired all the time and feeling cold. If that sounds familiar, do go to see your doctor and have yourself tested. Fluid retention can also make you gain weight and can be connected to the menstrual cycle or taking the Pill in women, or the use of corticosteroids. Again, a conversation with your doctor would probably be useful.*

51

Support act

Only you can lose your excess weight, but it's a whole lot easier if you have a support team to help. From formal support to the goodwill of family and friends, it's essential to feel you're not alone,

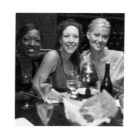

I don't like my partner to do the food shopping because he ignores my list. It is not his fault, it turns out — it is mine for not enlisting him as an ally. It's up to you to rally your supporters and keep them on side.

When my partner goes shopping, instead of bringing back lots of fruit and vegetables, low-fat dairy products, brown bread, rice and lean cuts of meat, he'll just bring a few of those, plus lots of 'extras' like full-fat cheeses, quiches, ice-cream and sausages. At first it was quite funny and endearing. Now it's getting expensive and annoying. I thought perhaps it was a deliberate ruse to get out of doing the supermarket run, but then I realised I'd never told him why I wanted the produce on the list and what wasn't good about all the fatty stuff he liked to bring back home.

'Ask your child what he wants for dinner only if he's buying.'
FRAN LEBOWITZ

Defining idea...

Improving your posture can make you look slimmer instantly. Relax your shoulders and draw them down and slightly back. Your chest should then naturally lift. Investigate Pilates or Alexander technique classes for more posture skills.

You've got to communicate your weight loss ambitions and plans to your partner and family. You need to sit them down and explain why you want to lose weight and also how you're going to go about it. It's important to ask for their help at this stage too. It could be for example that you'll need help with childcare, running errands, cooking or shopping. Perhaps you'd like them to exercise with you. Could they be eating more healthily too? If they're slim, they could eat the healthier foods you'll be choosing, but in larger quantities. If they're carrying a little excess baggage themselves, your motivation could well inspire them. At the very least the praise and encouragement of your nearest and dearest will be vital during your battle with the bulge.

Of course it's not unknown for those closest to you to be unenthusiastic, even obstructive, about you wanting to slim down. They're used to the cuddly you and fear that you'll change personality as well as size. Partners can harbour worries that the new slim you will run off with someone else. All you can do is be reassuring, but if they continue to be unsupportive, you'll just have to get on with it quietly. Try making new friends too. Meeting people in the same position as you is terrific for moral support. It's the contact and understanding that counts, not to mention the sharing of tips and advice.

'It is the friends you can call up at 4 a.m. that matter.'
MARLENE DIETRICH

As well as the support structure of family and friends, a more formal arrangement might suit you even better. Slimming clubs, such as WeightWatchers, Slimming World and Rosemary Conley have meetings nationwide, not to mention internet services and magazines. As well as the actual diets themselves, which are all basically healthy eating with slightly different approaches, the community spirit is great, high on support, motivation and inspiration. Research also confirms that your chances of losing weight and keeping it off are higher if you join a club.

Depending on your financial circumstances, you could also go for one-to-one help and support. A personal trainer could devise a tailor-made exercise plan for you and really help with your commitment to exercise – there's nothing like your personal trainer calling you through your letterbox to get you out of bed in the morning! You could also see a dietician for nutrition advice as well as ongoing support. There are diet coaches who are like life coaches but specialise in weight loss. They mostly work on the phone, though some do face-to-face as well. They are marvellous for helping you draw up an action plan and stick to it. Ultimately, it's your determination that will help you succeed, but you should also take all the help you can get.

Is it really a lack of support or just a handy excuse? Don't sabotage yourself! See IDEA 50, What's your excuse?

Try another idea...

'People change and forget to tell each other.'
LILLIAN HELLMAN

Defining idea...

227

How did it go?

Q **We have dinner with a couple we're friendly with quite often. She knows I'm trying to lose weight, but serves up really fatty foods. What should I do?**

A *Is she not thinking, or is she a bitch? If you enjoy their company, I'd attempt to grin and bear it and just eat small portions. Have a salad or bowl of soup before going over to their place. You have to be gracious and well-mannered, but that doesn't mean you can't pass up pudding: say the main course was so delicious and filling that you simply can't eat any more.*

Q **My partner and kids are overweight. How can I avoid giving the children a complex about weight issues?**

A *This is a tricky one, but to be blunt, obesity is a bigger problem for teenagers today than eating disorders. Seventy per cent of overweight teens grow into overweight adults. I think the way to deal with it is subtlety. Get more active as a family and make small changes in your eating habits. Cut down on junk and processed foods and swap to low fat dairy products and sugar free drinks and spreads. The fewer tempting snacks you have in the house, the less easy it is for them to grab one and slump in front of the TV. I'd also encourage them to learn more about food basics, either from websites such as the Food Standards Agency, the British Dietetic Association or food books. Kids enjoy learning; they may even end up teaching you a thing or two!*

52

Zen and the art of weight loss maintenance

We can all lose weight, at least in the short term, but the greatest challenge is keeping it off. What are the secrets of success?

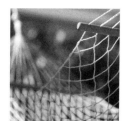

There's an often-quoted figure that 90% of people who lose weight put it all back on within a year. Estimates vary from 95 to 80%, but at any level above zero, it's too high.

However you look at it, there are a lot of people who don't keep up their weight loss. Rather than dwelling on the reasons for this 'failure', try to figure out how the 10, 5 or indeed 20% of people who have lost weight and kept it off have done it. Using studies, research and anecdotes, the reasons they succeed where others don't looks something like this:

Get a life! Successful dieters don't say 'When I lose weight, I'll take that holiday/get a new job/sort out my love life.' They just carry on with living alongside losing weight. So don't put your life on hold: do what you have to do and the rest will follow. It really will, honestly!

SUCCESS STRATEGY 1

People who keep weight off link their positive healthy behaviours with other areas of their lives. For instance, eating sensibly not only helps your health and weight, but it could set a good example to children. Exercise becomes not simply physical activity, but also a way of spending time with your partner, friends, kids and the dog! Many people also find that having started to take a real interest in nutrition and fitness for dieting reasons, they're inspired to build new careers as dieticians, fitness instructors and complementary medicine practitioners. Any change is great, but if it has a powerful effect on other areas of your life, it's more likely to stick.

SUCCESS STRATEGY 2

Small changes over a long period of time will become an integral part of your lifestyle, unlike short-termist tactics. Short-term plans only work in the short term, which is why for example crash dieting ultimately fails. Once you've lost your excess weight, the slimmer you will need fewer calories for maintenance. If you go back to your old eating habits, you'll put weight back on.

If your eating habits are changed gradually, you'll lose weight slowly and safely and the new habits will start to become second nature – the recipe for permanence.

SUCCESS STRATEGY 3

People who lose weight and keep it off know the value of exercise, combining both aerobic activity with resistance training. Not only does exercise help burn off calories – and fat if you do it for long enough – but it will also build muscle, which uses up more calories than fat does. It keeps you in shape from a health perspective too, protecting against osteoporosis, cardiovascular disease, high blood pressure and depression to name but a few. People who exercise also tend to have greater self-esteem than non-exercisers. As with healthy eating habits, exercise has to be consistent and regular to deliver benefits.

SUCCESS STRATEGY 4

Research has found that if your weight loss is motivated by health reasons, it's more likely to stay off long term than if it's motivated by looks alone.

SUCCESS STRATEGY 5

Long-term weight losers have also developed a well-balanced approach to food and themselves in relation to it. They know they can get themselves back on track if they gain weight and that is by forgiving themselves rather than dwelling on the potential consequences of eating another slice of chocolate cake. Ultimately the consistency (albeit with occasional lapses allowed) of eating low fat, low, but not too low, calorie, with a balance of protein, carbohydrates and plenty of fruit and vegetables is the eating pattern that generates long-term success.

Would a detox diet help you stay trim? See IDEA 20, *Detox diets – con or cure?*

Try another idea...

'Success is getting what you want. Happiness is wanting what you get.'
DALE CARNEGIE

Defining idea...

How did it go?

Q I've heard about a 'set point' theory that we all have a natural weight which you can't change. Is this true?

A   *It is a theory and it's still being debated. The idea is if you lose weight below your set point, your body will do everything it can to get you back to your former weight – it could explain why so many of us find weight loss hard to maintain. How annoying it is that the theory doesn't work in reverse – if you put too much weight on, your body doesn't fight to get it off! Even if it is found to be true, exercise is still the way to regain control as it can raise your metabolism and encourages fat to be used up.*

Q Can I lose weight without dieting – say with exercise alone?

A   *Yes, you can lose weight just with a regular exercise routine, as long as you don't also eat more. To lose a significant amount you'd have to work out hard. I suggest you get a trainer in your local gym or health club to help you devise a programme, but you could also achieve a slower loss over time by burning up just a few hundred calories extra a day than you currently do. However, just because you burn off your calories doesn't mean you're well-nourished. It's important to eat healthily too!*

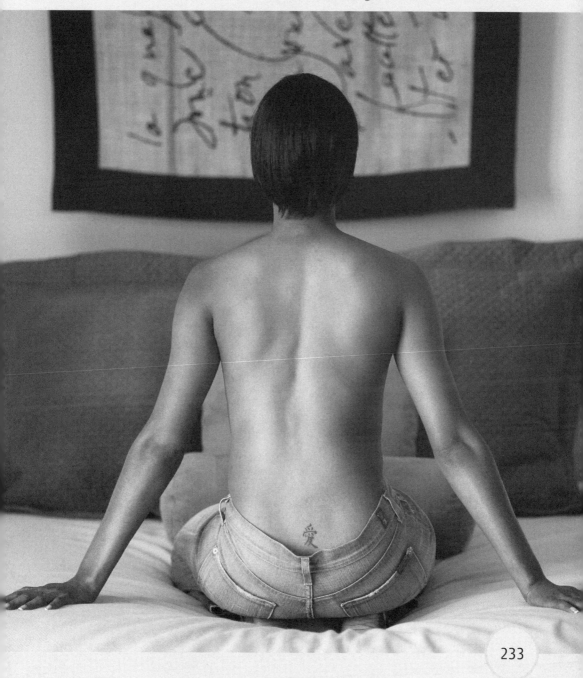

The end...

Or is it a new beginning?

We hope that the ideas in this book will have inspired you to try some new things. You should be well on your way to a slimmer you. And you can look also forward to a healthier, fitter, more fulfilled and balanced you, brimming with good intentions.

You're mean, you're motivated and you don't care who knows it.

So why not let *us* know all about it? Tell us how you got on. What did it for you – what helped you beat the cravings? What got you back on your bike after years of motoring? Maybe you've got some tips of your own you want to share (see next page if so). And if you liked this book you may find we have even more brilliant ideas that could change other areas of your life for the better.

You'll find the Infinite Ideas crew waiting for you online at www.infideas.com.

Or if you prefer to write, then send your letters to:
Lose weight and stay slim
The Infinite Ideas Company Ltd
Belsyre Court, 57 Woodstock Road, Oxford OX2 6HJ, United Kingdom

We want to know what you think, because we're all working on making our lives better too. Give us your feedback and you could win a copy of another *52 Brilliant Ideas* book of your choice. Or maybe get a crack at writing your own.

Good luck. Be brilliant.

Offer one

CASH IN YOUR IDEAS

We hope you enjoy this book. We hope it inspires, amuses, educates and entertains you. But we don't assume that you're a novice, or that this is the first book that you've bought on the subject. You've got ideas of your own. Maybe our author has missed an idea that you use successfully. If so, why not send it to info@infideas.com, and if we like it we'll post it on our bulletin board. Better still, if your idea makes it into print we'll send you £50 and you'll be fully credited so that everyone knows you've had another Brilliant Idea.

Offer two

HOW COULD YOU REFUSE?

Amazing discounts on bulk quantities of Infinite Ideas books are available to corporations, professional associations and other organizations.

For details call us on:
+44 (0)1865 292045
fax: +44 (0)1865 292001
or e-mail: info@infideas.com

235

Where it's at...